THE
GREAT
PLAGUE

THE
GREAT
PLAGUE

STEPHEN
PORTER

SUTTON PUBLISHING

First published in 1999 by
Sutton Publishing Limited · Phoenix Mill
Thrupp · Stroud · Gloucestershire · GL5 2BU

British Library Cataloguing in Publication Data
A catalogue record for this book is available from the British Library

ISBN 0 7509 1615 X

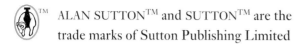

ALAN SUTTON™ and SUTTON™ are the
trade marks of Sutton Publishing Limited

Typeset in 11/15pt Ehrhardt.
Typesetting and origination by
Sutton Publishing Limited.
Printed in Great Britain by
Redwood, Trowbridge, Wiltshire.

3/00

Contents

List of Illustrations

Acknowledgements

Plague has been a topic of enduring interest, both in the period when it was active in western Europe and since. This interest has generated a considerable literature, and I have much appreciated the labours of numerous authors and editors whose work I have drawn upon in preparing this book. The interpretations within it are, of course, my own.

I am most grateful to the Governors of Sutton's Hospital in Charterhouse for allowing me access to their archives, and to Gordon Forster, Adam White and Gary Tuson of Derbyshire Record Office, for dealing with my queries. Having tolerated civil war and fire, my colleagues have now shown great forbearance with my preoccupation with a topic which may not be entirely central to their own interests. Ann Robey, John Bold, Derek Kendall, June Warrington, Derek Kendall, George Wilson and Harriet Richardson have been especially helpful. Michael Clements prepared the figures.

Writing a book on such a potentially melancholy topic requires a cheerful context, and this was provided by my wife Carolyn, who also gave much helpful advice, combined with her usual challenging comments.

CHAPTER 1

Plague and Society

Friar John: One of our order, to associate me,
   Here in this city visiting the sick,
   And finding him, the searchers of the town,
   Suspecting that we both were in a house
   Where the infectious pestilence did reign,
   Seal'd up the doors, and would not let us forth

William Shakespeare, *Romeo and Juliet*, V. ii

Because of Friar John's confinement in the house in Verona he was unable to deliver a message to Romeo at Mantua. The message explained that news of Juliet's death was false, for she had taken a potion to render her insensible for a time, to avoid marriage to Paris. His failure to deliver this information was crucial, for Romeo did indeed hear of her death and, unaware of the circumstances, returned in anguish to Verona. From that point the tragedy unfolded inexorably. Shakespeare's audiences would immediately have understood his device, for plague intermittently disrupted social and commercial intercourse, as it had been doing for almost 250 years.

When the chronicler Henry Knighton described the origins of the Black Death in the 1340s, he noted that it had begun in India, spreading from there to Asia Minor and then infecting the Christian and Jewish populations.[1] From its first arrival in Europe at the Sicilian city of Messina in October 1347, the plague rapidly dispersed through Italy and then across much of the continent, reaching England in the following year. The speed with which it advanced, its contagiousness, the high mortality rate among those who contracted it, the large numbers of its victims, the failure to check its progress or to devise a cure and the sheer foulness of the illness made it the most feared of all the diseases that afflicted late medieval and early modern Europe. Its prominence in this respect was reflected in the fact that it was often referred to simply as 'the sickness' or 'the pestilence'. Western Europe had been free from the disease between the

Plague of Justinian in the sixth and seventh centuries and the Black Death, but from the 1340s until the 1720s it was subject to periodic epidemics of plague of varying intensity and extent, some striking a relatively restricted area, others spreading over several countries.

The plague made an enormous impact on Europe, not only on its economy and society, but also upon its beliefs, literature and art. Populations were drastically reduced in a short space of time, social contacts broke down, household and community economies were disrupted or even wrecked, and both local and regional trade was interrupted as fear of outsiders bringing contagion outweighed economic needs. An individual's careful planning for the future might be completely nullified by an epidemic, which could wipe out entire families. The prospect of sudden death was an alarming one, not allowing the victims time to make proper provision, either for their possessions or their souls. Everyone seemed to be at risk from an eruption of the plague and the likelihood of dying a spiritual death, as well as a bodily one, with the soul sent abruptly to judgement without due preparation.[2] It appeared to be impossible to prevent the disease; even Sir Thomas More's perfectly regulated Utopia had twice been subjected to 'a great pestilential plague'.[3]

In the *Decameron*, Boccaccio described the effect which the Black Death had on Florence, where more than half the population may have perished in the epidemic of 1348.[4] He noted that almost all of the victims died within three days of the appearance of the swellings, or buboes, in the groin or armpit which characterised the disease. He commented, too, on the speed with which the infection spread through the population. It seemed that it could be caught simply by conversing with someone who was afflicted. Indeed, the plague was so virulent that contact with its victims was not necessary, for it could be contracted by handling their belongings. Just touching their clothes could prove fatal. He cited the story of pigs who, scavenging in the street, died shortly after tossing about some rags that had belonged to a poor victim of the disease.

The physicians proved to be helpless and unable to offer any effective treatment or preventive measures. In the panic caused by the epidemic, their failure permitted many who had no medical training to set themselves up as would-be doctors, offering quack remedies to the anxious Florentines. In the belief that the disease was carried on tainted air, a common safeguard was to carry nosegays of flowers or herbs that would ward off the foul vapours.

With the widespread fear caused by the virulent nature of the infection and the very high mortality rate among those who contracted the disease, the normal

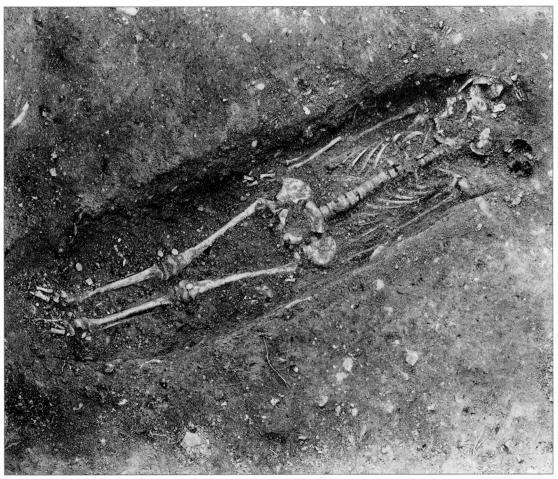

This skeleton of a child was uncovered on the site of the Black Death burial ground at Charterhouse Square, London. (© Crown copyright, NMR)

social practices associated with nursing the sick and burying the dead all but broke down. Victims were often deserted by almost everyone during their brief illness, including their relatives. Servants may have stayed on to attend to those who were ill, but that often cost them their lives. The sick were glad to have anyone to care for them and, contrary to convention, a woman did not object to being nursed by a man and was prepared to abandon her customary modesty.

Some victims died alone and unnoticed, and their corpses were detected only by the stench of their decaying. Not only were attempts at providing a dignified end for the mortally ill neglected, but the burial rites, too, were practically abandoned. In normal times the funeral procession would have been accompanied by members of the deceased's family, the neighbours and friends, yet during the epidemic no more than a dozen took part, and they were 'not the honourable or respected citizens'. In fact, those who went with the body were mostly poorer people acting as bearers rather than mourners. So many were dying or being taken ill that it became common to see the dead and sick being carried through the streets. Burial services were not observed at the church of the deceased's choice, but at the nearest or most convenient one, and the corpse was interred wherever a space could be found. Given the large numbers of deaths, the consecrated burial grounds were quickly filled and new, mass, graves had to be dug in order to dispose of the corpses.

The impression that the social order was under severe strain came partly from such curtailment of the usual burial rituals and partly from the behaviour of some sections of society. Boccaccio described how many of those who had been excluded from the city for criminal or social offences now returned, as the enforcement of such regulations disintegrated and the priorities of the administration shifted to deal with the current emergency. They now roamed around the streets in groups 'with riotous antics'. Indeed, with everyone remaining in the city living under a threat of imminent death, the poor were no longer bound by the usual social conventions and respectable citizens found themselves taunted with scurrilous songs.

Showing an apparent contempt for the danger by behaving in a carefree way was not confined to the poor. Boccaccio identified four typical reactions to the danger. Some citizens took few or no precautions to protect themselves from the plague, defying the risk of infection by mixing freely with others and gathering in groups at inns or taverns, drinking and revelling. Even members of the monastic orders gave themselves over to such riotous living. Other Florentines took a completely opposite course, living secluded lives, doing everything in moderation and listening to music to take their minds off the disaster unfolding around them. A third response was to take a middle course between these extremes, not becoming reclusive, but behaving cautiously when in public places. Finally, some citizens decided that the only way to avoid the epidemic was to leave the city. Even then, they had to be cautious about their choice of refuge, for the countryside was not free from plague. But flight was not an option that was available to many of the poorer and middling inhabitants, and they died in their homes in large numbers.

Many of the effects of the plague on mid-fourteenth century Florence can be recognised in the reactions to the epidemics that erupted throughout Europe

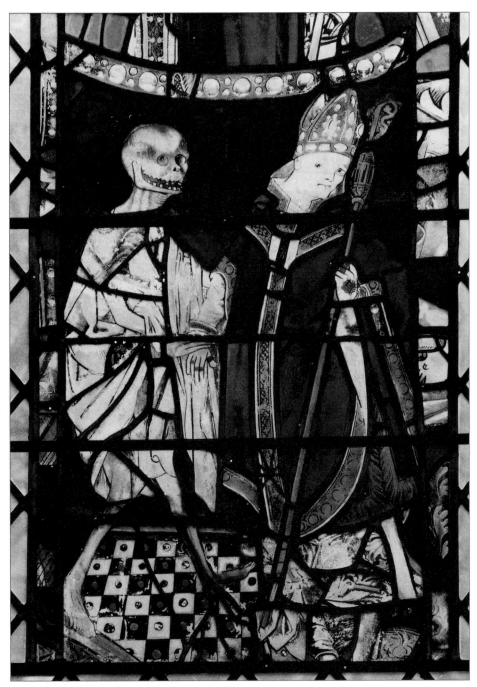

In this late fifteenth-century window at St Andrew's Church, Norwich, the reactions of the players suggest that the bishop has lost his game of checkers with the devil. No one was immune from plague, which brought sudden death and sent the soul on its journey unprepared.
(© Crown copyright, NMR)

until the early eighteenth century. Among them was the variation in death rates between the social classes. Obviously, the wealthier citizens were those who were most able to leave and stay away for the duration of the outbreak; for economic reasons the poorer people simply could not leave, and had to take their chances. Their predicament was succinctly described by John Hooper, Bishop of Gloucester in the 1550s, who wrote that 'there be certain persons that cannot flee although they would: as the poorer sort of people that have no friends nor place to flee unto, more than the poor house they dwell in'.[5] Partly for this reason, plague came to be regarded as a threat to the poor rather than to the whole population, and the districts in which they lived were seen as the breeding grounds for the disease. Plague thus brought into sharp focus a more fundamental division between rich and poor than material wealth and status, and social discontent became a common feature of epidemics, reflected not just in insulting behaviour, but in the looting of properties left empty by those who had fled. The abandonment of elaborate burial rituals – as the numbers of dead and need for

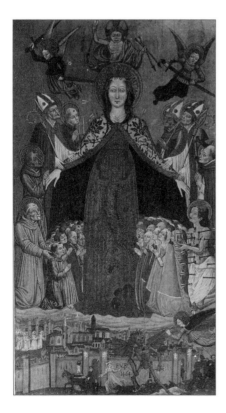

Benedetto Bonfigli's Gonfalone di San Francesco al Prato *of 1464 shows the plague demon bringing death to Perugia. The holy family departs unscathed and God sends his angels to end the city's sufferings.* (© Galleria Nazionale dell'Umbria)

speedy interment took priority over the normal arrangements – and the emergence of groups of people who were able to deal with the victims, were further characteristics of outbreaks of plague. While no preventive medicine or cure was developed, the practice of selling nosegays of concoctions to ward off the evil air that was thought to carry the disease continued, and the apothecaries were one group who could benefit from an outbreak.

Boccaccio was concerned chiefly with describing the awful effects of the plague on his city. He had little to say about the cause of the outbreak, other than to ascribe it to the influence of heavenly bodies or to divine wrath. Other writers thought that planetary activity had caused the corruption of the atmosphere, while one observer attributed it to the great earthquakes of 1347, which had released poisonous fumes into the air. To the Perugian artist Benedetto Bonfigli, the plague was a winged demon, with a body so decayed as to be virtually a skeleton, equipped with bow, arrows and quiver. Standing astride his victims outside the walls of the city, which suffered badly in an epidemic in 1464, he could be driven off only by an angel armed with a spear. Just seven years later Bonfigli depicted the plague not as the work of a demon, but as the vengeful hand of Christ, unleashing thunderbolts on the wicked city, while the Virgin and Saints intercede on Perugia's behalf.[6]

These continued to be common interpretations as plague epidemics repeatedly struck Europe in the late medieval and early modern periods. The outbreaks were seen as the product of some malign influence, or the vengeance inflicted by a wrathful God on a sinful and unrepentant population. Divine anger for misdeeds was a familiar explanation for all illness, not just the plague, and this persisted in being the interpretation, even in the Protestant regions of northern Europe after the Reformation. The logical conclusion to be drawn from this assumption was that an epidemic was not a chance event with natural causes, but a working out of God's purpose. It may have been provoked by any number of a range of sins or the toleration by society of ungodly groups. In the context of post-Reformation England these included Roman Catholics, nonconformists, foreigners, sabbath-breakers, prostitutes and theatre-goers. Such tolerance would explain why the plague was so widespread, and not an affliction borne only by the offending categories or by even smaller groups, such as particularly sinful families or the regular frequenters of alehouses. Similarly, the severe outbreaks in England in 1603 and 1625, with high mortality in London in both years, coincided with a change of monarch and were interpreted as a need for the population to be purged of the sins of the previous reign.[7] But an outbreak of plague could also be seen not only as a punishment for past sins, but as a warning, a call to repent and reform. Attempts could be made to assuage God's anger by penitence and fasting, and by dealing with those groups who were assumed to have given offence.

In addition to an anxiety to explain the causes of plague, there was a need for accurate predictions of future epidemics. Patterns were sought in the occurrences of past outbreaks. When no epidemics struck after the death of Charles I in 1649 or the restoration of the monarchy with Charles II in 1660, the theory that plague came at the change of reign took a serious knock. Nor did the contention that an epidemic came every twenty years stand serious examination, although it was widely accepted. Visionary preachers and writers were able to provide terrifying images of a future visitation, with Thomas Reeve in 1657 predicting that 'there will then be no other music to be heard but dolefull knells, nor no other wares to be borne up and down but dead corpses'.[8] But they were less forthcoming about when the next such disaster would occur. This was more the province of the astrologers. On the basis that a malign conjunction of the stars, especially of Saturn and Mars, could result in the atmospheric corruption associated with plague, they cast a city's horoscope to predict future epidemics. By the mid-seventeenth century this practice had become a relatively common one.[9]

The assumption that an epidemic was caused by God's wrath or the movements of the heavenly bodies could lead to fatalism. Furthermore, awareness of the variable social impact of plague may have produced a certain complacency, for those who were able to do so could leave a stricken community and survive, while 'the poorer and meaner sort', who could not, were 'not of such use, but may better be spared'.[10] The crowded and dirty living conditions of the poor, perhaps also their corrupt diet, could be seen as the reasons for their suffering. So, too, could their lack of care during an outbreak of plague, which verged on the recklessness noted by Boccaccio, despite the obvious risk of disease and probably death. Given such behaviour, it may have seemed that nothing could be done to limit the scale of a disaster. Perhaps the plague was a divine instrument for reducing the population, with the poor the chief sufferers because, as the warden of the pest-house at Genoa in the plague years of the 1650s suggested, they had failed to restrict their marriages, unlike the richer citizens.[11]

Yet throughout the period, and in parts of Italy from the onset of the Black Death in the 1340s, practical measures were adopted to prevent outbreaks of plague, by dealing with their presumed causes, and to reduce their impact if they did occur. Those who attempted to tackle the problem had much opportunity to observe the disease and its characteristics, for epidemics, albeit irregular, were

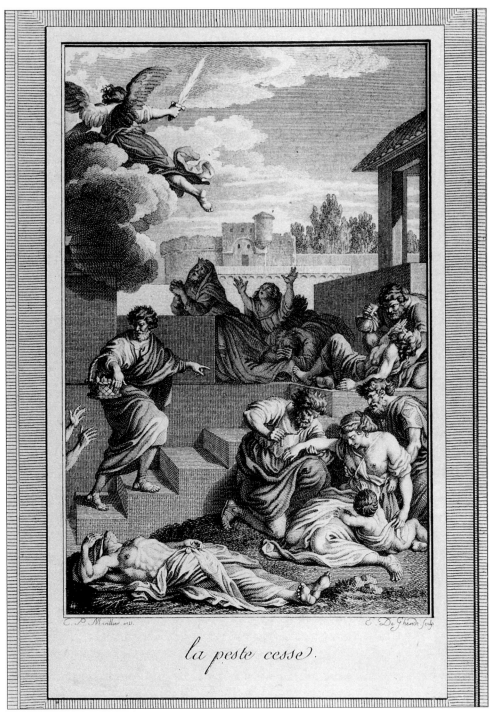

la peste cesse.

Clément-Pierre Marillier's La Peste Cesse *shows the angel of God intervening to halt the plague. An etching by E. de Ghendt.* (© The Wellcome Institute Library, London)

relatively frequent. A basic assumption underlying the measures taken to prevent plague was that wholesome air could be corrupted by decaying rubbish and turned into miasmic, or poisonous, air, which provided the ideal environment for the venomous atoms that brought the disease. The atoms would adhere to any object, animal or person, although they were more likely to stick to a rough surface, such as that provided by wool or cloth, than a smooth one. A part of the solution was to prevent the vapours that caused the unwholesome air from forming, by creating a cleaner environment.

Boccaccio mentioned that steps had been taken in Florence to cleanse the city and prevent the sick from being admitted. Such restriction of movement and quarantining of travellers and goods from places known or suspected to have plague was one stratagem that was widely adopted. Quarantine regulations were put in place at Dubrovnik in 1465 and at Venice in 1485. An associated measure was the issue of passes to those wishing to travel, certifying that the bearer had come from a place that was free of plague, or had not been in contact with a victim. Travellers had to renew their *Bolletino della sanità* at every town. The isolation of the sick within the community was also common. This was done by confining them to their homes and forbidding them to have visitors, or by moving them into pest-houses that stood apart from other buildings and keeping them there for a specified period. Fear that goods, especially textiles, could spread the plague led to the provision of buildings where they could be fumigated and held in quarantine. A pest-house for silks was set up in Tuscany in 1631.[12]

The segregation of large numbers of plague suspects required the founding or rebuilding of hospitals and pest-houses. The earliest case of an isolation hospital was that built at Venice in 1403, while the best known and perhaps most widely admired was the 1488 Lazaretto di San Gregorio at Milan. Its design resembled that of a Carthusian priory, with a large rectangular courtyard ringed by individual cells in which the patients could be kept in isolation. It was on a far larger scale than any monastic house, however, for the courtyard was 413 yd by 405 yd, with 288 cells. During an epidemic temporary huts could be built in the courtyard and 16,000 patients were said to have been accommodated there during the plague of 1630. John Evelyn visited the hospital in 1646 and described it admiringly as 'a quadrangular Cloyster, of a vast compasse: in earnest a royal fabric'.[13] The pest-house at Genoa was also a large and impressive one. When it was inspected in 1652 German mercenaries were keeping guard there and 293 patients were being held in quarantine, while the two main hospitals in the city contained a further 1,114 patients.[14]

Such hospitals were designed on a scale that could deal with the numbers stricken during the intermittent plague outbreaks, but they could, of course, be used for nursing the sick in normal times, and pest-houses could provide shelter for the homeless poor in non-plague years. Similarly, the regulations that were concerned with public health included those which related specifically to outbreaks of plague, such as ensuring that corpses were buried promptly and at an adequate depth, and others which remained in force when there was no epidemic. In the belief that humans could catch the plague from infected animals, when an outbreak threatened cats and dogs were killed in large numbers. Gatherings of people were banned and institutions such as schools and almshouses temporarily closed and their inmates either confined within the buildings or sent away.

Many of the increasingly wide-ranging controls that were imposed, even during the periods when there was no perceptible danger from plague, attempted to deal with the threat apparently posed by dirt and smells. They were designed to enforce cleanliness, by overseeing the paving of streets and market-places, the removal of putrefying rubbish and manure, sanitary conditions in inns and the quality of food for sale. Such health and hygiene measures came to be regulated by boards of health and health officers. As early as March 1348 Venice appointed a committee of three men to maintain public health in the face of the imminent threat of the Black Death. In the fourteenth century such boards generally continued only during epidemics, or until the danger had passed, but in the fifteenth and sixteenth centuries they came increasingly to be established as permanent bodies. Magistracies for health matters were set up in Milan during the first half of the fifteenth century, at Venice in 1486, at Florence in 1527 and at Lucca in 1549. Many other places in northern and central Italy followed, and by the second half of the sixteenth century all of the principal cities had appointed such a board, and some smaller towns and villages also had health boards or officers. Their competence extended to the supervision of the medical profession, the care of the sick and the administration of hospitals.[15]

In order to have effective controls in place as soon as possible when an epidemic threatened, the causes of death were recorded. A death certificate was required, signed by a doctor or surgeon. From the statistics, the numbers dying from plague, and indeed from other diseases, could be identified, and the beginnings of an outbreak recognised. The process was initiated at Milan in 1452 and a continuous sequence of such *Bills of Mortality* for the city survives from 1503, while the *Bills* for Mantua begin in 1496, for Venice in 1504 and for Modena in 1554.[16]

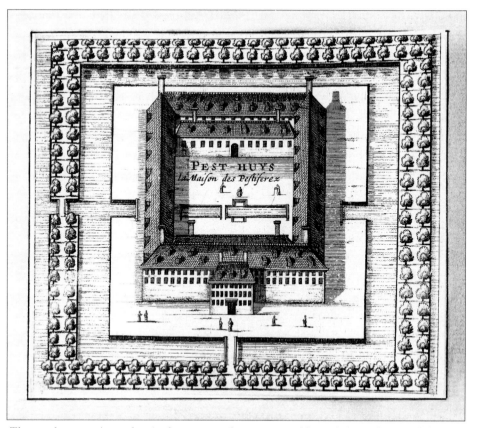

The pest-house at Amsterdam in the seventeenth century stood beyond the city's outer defences. (© The Wellcome Institute Library, London)

By the mid-seventeenth century Italy was regarded as 'the strictest place in the world, in the case of health', and many of the measures taken there to combat plague had been adopted quite widely in western Europe.[17] They were common solutions to a common problem, arrived at both locally and by imitation of those employed elsewhere. Quarantine stations were erected at Marseilles in 1383 and plague regulations were introduced at Troyes in 1517, Reims in 1522 and Paris in 1531, where a public health officer was appointed in 1580, a year of epidemic.[18] At Amsterdam rubbish removal services were put in place in the 1590s and the health establishment included a plague doctor. The city's pest-house was a substantial courtyard building standing in an undeveloped area beyond the outer defences and enclosed by canals, and with a channel running through the building. An epidemic at Zwolle in 1655 prompted the town council to establish a 'plague advisory body', which set up a special hospital.[19] Delft had a plague hospital in the buildings of the former convent of Maria Magdalen from before the Reformation until they were destroyed in the explosion of 1654. A replacement was then built outside the centre of the town.[20]

The expense of supporting the sick became a major problem during epidemics, taking almost all of the city's revenues at Montpellier in 1530, and compelling the magistrat at Lille to impose extra taxes during epidemics in the late 1550s and again in 1575, to cover the cost of maintaining those confined at home or in the quarantine barracks outside the city walls.[21] Nevertheless, despite the recurrent outbreaks of plague, the implementation of steps to ameliorate its impact often took time. The need for a plague hospital at Paris was recognised as early as 1496, but not until 1580 was one begun, based on the hospital at Milan, and the incomplete buildings were demolished a few years later. Only with the building of L'Hôpital St Louis between 1607 and 1612 was the city's need for such a hospital realised.[22]

Physical separation from the continent did not give the British Isles immunity from plague, in the seventh century, during the Black Death, or later. Indeed, the frequency of outbreaks and seasonality of deaths suggest that the disease was endemic throughout the later Middle Ages.[23] Epidemics struck repeatedly, with at least eighteen which can be classed as being national in scale between 1348 and 1485. Colchester experienced high mortality in nine of the thirty years after 1410, while, at a more local level, the obituary lists for Christ Church priory in Canterbury show that deaths from plague occurred in thirteen of the years between 1413 and 1517, and that the disease accounted for 41 of the 254 deaths there during that period.[24] As both national and urban populations began to rise from the late fifteenth century, plague continued to take a heavy toll. Epidemics struck Gloucester in nine of the last thirty-five years of the sixteenth century, and Norwich endured severe outbreaks in 1579–80, 1584–5 and 1589–92.[25] Although the greatest impact was on towns, rural communities were by no means immune. During an epidemic in Devon from 1589 to 1591, burials in seventeen country parishes across the county were on average more than five times their normal level. Even a remote settlement such as Widecombe-in-the-Moor was affected, with sixty-eight burials in 1590–1, compared with an annual average of fewer than twenty.[26]

The epidemics of the sixteenth and seventeenth centuries erupted against a background of an emerging national policy aimed at combating the disease. Its beginnings can be seen in the measures set out in a royal proclamation of 1518, which ordered that houses in London where the infection had been recognised should have bundles of straw hanging from their windows so that they could be identified, and their occupants should carry white sticks when they went out. These orders were promulgated in Oxford in the same year, on the prompting of Sir Thomas More, and were similar to those issued in Paris in 1510. Also in 1518, the Royal College of Physicians was founded, and five years later its licensing powers over the profession were extended from London to the whole of England.[27]

By the middle of the sixteenth century the isolation of the sick had been widely adopted as a means of limiting the spread of an outbreak of plague. The Privy Council was clear that it was not the 'corruption of the air' that caused the disease to spread, but the failure to quarantine those who were infected, and their unwillingness to isolate themselves. From marking their houses with bundles of straw, the Council came to prefer a cross and the words 'Lord Have Mercy Upon Us'. Confinement was attempted by preventing occupants from leaving their houses, or by compelling them to move to pest-houses that were, ideally at least, placed on the edge of a town. The problem with pest-houses was their limited capacity, causing the magistrates at Gloucester and Leicester to adopt the more drastic solution of sealing off a district where plague had broken out. The implication of confining the sick, however it was attempted, was that they needed practical support, especially a dependable supply of food, if they were not to suffer distress and even starvation. Without such support the orders were bound to be difficult to enforce. Charitable donations and the provisions brought by relatives and friends were too uncertain. This problem was addressed by the magistrates at York in 1550 when they introduced a weekly rate to maintain those in quarantine, a practice that was soon imitated elsewhere.[28]

Other steps taken when an outbreak threatened included orders that the streets be cleaned and piles of rubbish removed, that animals should not be taken through the streets, that the admission of visitors to a town should be strictly controlled, and that goods from places known to be infected should be prohibited. Gatherings of people at feasts, weddings or funerals were banned, travelling players were prohibited from performing, theatres were closed and, if the danger was thought to be serious enough, markets and fairs were cancelled, despite the economic damage that ensued. If an epidemic did begin, then searchers and other officials were appointed who were responsible for identifying the sick, organising the burial of the dead and the cleaning of infected houses. In 1584 the vestry of the London parish of St Andrew, Holborn, listed the personnel required as 'viewers, searchers, keepers, watchers, surveyors, collectors, providers, deliverers, and such like officers'.[29] Burials were to be held only at specified times during the hours of darkness and the number of mourners was limited. Animals were to be kept indoors – stray dogs and cats were killed, because they were suspected of being carriers of plague – and fires were lit in the streets to dispel the foul air.[30] These measures were introduced in many towns during the second half of the sixteenth century, especially during the 1570s. Increasingly, corporations issued codifications of plague orders as the disease threatened, signifying a more coherent and orderly response to the problem than the earlier piecemeal and often sluggish reactions.

To provide warning of a threatened outbreak and allow measures to be put in place to check its progress, *Bills of Mortality* were introduced, based upon the Italian models. The earliest London *Bill* was compiled in 1519, and they were prepared in other years of epidemic during the early sixteenth century, plague deaths being distinguished from the others. In 1555 the parish clerks were instructed to make a return of 'the numbers of all the persons who die and whereof they die'. The weekly returns for London were printed from the early 1610s onwards, making them widely available, and they not only became more sophisticated, distinguishing a range of causes of death, but they were issued until the mid-nineteenth century, long after the final outbreak of plague. Some provincial towns, such as Norwich, Bristol, Chester and York, also came to record such statistics.[31]

London presented a greater problem than the provincial towns, partly because of its sheer size and seemingly inexorable growth, and partly because of the different authorities responsible for its government. The corporation administered the City itself, but the expanding suburbs north of the river came under the jurisdiction of the Middlesex justices, and Southwark under the Surrey ones. In addition, London attracted much closer attention from the government than any other city, because of its role as national capital, its economic importance and its proximity to the royal court at Whitehall.

The capital's population grew from around 120,000 in 1550 to 200,000 in 1600 and then doubled to at least 400,000 by the middle of the seventeenth century. Within the metropolis, the proportion of the City's population fell steadily, for much of the growth was in the suburbs, especially those north of the Thames. In 1580 the City contained almost three-quarters of the inhabitants, yet by 1640 fewer than 40 per cent lived within the corporation's jurisdiction.[32] This caused considerable anxiety, not only because of the increasing numbers flocking to the capital, but also as a result of the poor quality of the buildings erected to house them and the environment that was created. The suburbs came to be seen as foul and polluted, producing the very conditions in which it was thought that plague could thrive. When the Elizabethan and early Stuart governments attempted to curb the growth of London, they cited the risk of plague as one of the reasons for their action. The proclamation of 1603 specifically attributed the epidemic of that year to the 'pestering of excessive numbers of idle, indigent, dissolute and dangerous persons in small and strait rooms and habitations'. Reflecting such concerns, the Commission for New Buildings, created in 1618, dealt with a wider range of matters than its name would suggest, including environmental conditions, such as improved sewage disposal arrangements.[33]

The Privy Council acted from time to time to stimulate the corporation's efforts regarding plague, as in 1543 when it directed the Lord Mayor to draw up precepts and articles, which were to be passed to the aldermen. Yet the response was often lethargic. Indeed, the absence of an effective strategy that should be implemented when a crisis threatened was highlighted by the devastating epidemic of 1563. Fires were lit in the streets, dogs were killed and crosses were fixed to the houses of the victims, but no financial provision was made and so the quarantining of suspected cases was impossible to enforce. Not until the Privy Council intervened early in 1564, when the worst was over, was isolation implemented. Additional measures were devised following that outbreak and a less severe one in 1570, and in 1574 the orders were printed and posted up in the streets. Eventually, in 1583 a set of twenty-one orders was issued, and this formed the basis of the London plague orders that were produced until the Great Plague of 1665. These largely followed existing practices, specifying such measures as the isolation of the sick, cleaning of the streets, the expulsion of vagrants and prohibitions of public gatherings.[34]

Before the London orders were codified, in 1578 the Privy Council had devised a set of seventeen orders 'to be executed throughout the Counties of this Realm in such . . . places as are . . . infected with the plague'. As with those issued by the corporation, they were to be repeated largely unchanged until 1665. Among the measures included in the national plague orders was one which finally resolved the question of how long the quarantine for infected houses should last, by specifying a period of six weeks. Furthermore, the quarantine was to be strictly enforced for all members of the household and the Plague Act of 1604 empowered the watchmen to use force to ensure that it was not broken. The orders also stipulated that taxes to maintain the sick should be levied during epidemics, thereby not leaving it to local magistrates to decide whether to impose them or not.[35] Here at last was a national policy aimed at minimising the extent of plague and dealing with its consequences. Yet on two important points the City resisted the Privy Council's promptings. Firstly, it insisted that it could not afford to maintain the large body of officials required to implement the orders, hence a smaller complement was approved. Because of this, a concession had to be made in the orders by permitting one member of an isolated household to leave the building to get food. Complete segregation was not specified in London until 1608. Secondly, the City objected to the raising of a compulsory plague rate, preferring charitable collections and the existing rates for poor relief.[36]

Financial concerns also delayed the building of a pest-house in the capital. Although urged by the Privy Council in 1583 to erect such a building, as had been done in 'many cities of less antiquity, fame, wealth, circuit and reputation', work did not begin until 1594. The pest-house stood in the parish of St Giles, Cripplegate and may not have been large enough to hold more than 200 or 300 suspected plague victims at a time. In 1638 a pest-house was built in Tothill Fields, Westminster, but that seems to have been an insubstantial structure, referred to as 'the sheds'.[37] During an epidemic the accommodation was supplemented by temporary cabins, the solution also adopted by many provincial towns.

The coherent policy that emerged during Elizabeth's reign was continued throughout the first half of the seventeenth century, albeit with some modifications and additions. When royal proclamations were issued in 1607 and 1610 to limit starch making, they cited the stench produced by the process as 'no small cause of the breeding and nourishing of the plague'. This contradicted the Privy Council's earlier view, expressed in 1578, that the disease was spread by failure to isolate the victims, not by foul air.[38] In fact, the miasmic explanation of plague was still a popular one. Because of the risk of contagion, in 1606 Hull corporation ordered that the keeping and curing of fish-livers should not take place within half a mile of the town.[39] The absorbent powers of onions were recommended for collecting the infection, and the belief that they could be used as an indicator of the presence of plague, by changing colour, was ridiculed by Ben Jonson in *Volpone*. During one of the major London epidemics in the early seventeenth century someone allegedly had the idea of filling a ship with peeled onions and, when the wind direction was favourable, floating it down the Thames through the capital. The air pollution would then be attracted to the onions and thus carried away on the ship to the North Sea. After mentioning how much mirth the story had caused, John Evelyn went on to recommend the creation around London of plantations of fragrant shrubs and other plants, to improve the air.[40] The plague orders of 1592 advised burning a concoction of herbs and carrying the smouldering mixture from room to room to purify a building. During the London plague of 1593 the actor Edward Alleyn advised his wife to throw water outside the door and to line the windows with a 'good store of rue and herb of grace'. Individuals continued to seek protection from the plague by carrying nosegays, sprigs of rosemary, rue, or other sweet-smelling herbs, and, as smoking became more common, by puffing a pipe of tobacco. Apothecaries doubtless tailored their potions to the means of the client. In 1607 the Earl of Northumberland paid 10s for a pomander, and £5 for a pair of rubies.[41]

When a severe epidemic threatened to erupt in London in 1630, as it did over much of Europe, the government asked both the College of Physicians and Sir Theodore de Mayerne, the king's physician, for guidance. Among the reasons for plague, the College pointed to overcrowded housing, the large number of burials in churches, the interment of plague victims in churches and churchyards, and bad meat and rotten fish. They also drew attention to poor standards of cleanliness, such as the failure to clean ditches and sewers, dirty streets, ponds of standing water at inns, the presence of laystalls near the city and of slaughter houses within it. Mayerne agreed that overcrowding was one of the problems, as were poor vagrants. His recommendations included the creation of a board of health for London, and perhaps in provincial cities, and the erection of four or five pest-houses in the capital, including a plague hospital, the model for which was clearly L'Hôpital St Louis in Paris. Parishes were to be combined to form five districts, each having staff such as apothecaries and searchers. The numbers of taverns, alehouses and tobacco shops were to be reduced and premises producing offensive smells, such as slaughter houses, fishmarkets and tanneries, were to be removed from the city. Rubbish removal and the cleanliness of ditches were to be improved, foul alleys were to be cleared of their population and perhaps pulled down, and stray cats and dogs were to be killed. So, too, were rats, mice and weasels, because in their moving about and going from house to house they may contract and transmit the infection. For much of his proposed programme, Mayerne clearly drew on his experience of the Paris of Henri IV, but Italy was the model for his suggestion that shipping coming from abroad at a time of contagion ought to produce certificates of clean health and that their crews and passengers should be quarantined for forty days.[42]

Quarantining of shipping had been employed on a number of earlier occasions and was again applied by a royal proclamation of 1635, prompted by plague in France and the Low Countries. This ordered that a certificate had to be obtained from the customs officers before the crew or passengers were allowed to disembark or goods could be landed, assuming that the place of origin was free from the disease. If the vessel or its cargo came from somewhere that was suspect, a quarantine of twenty days should be enforced.[43]

Mayerne's suggestions for a hospital, boards of health and extra pest-houses in London were not implemented, and other elements in his programme and the submission by the College of Physicians were already a part of the established policy for plague. The need to clean the streets and prevent the accumulation of piles of manure and other rubbish was recognised in many towns, with scavengers appointed for the purpose. Even so, the responsibility for keeping the streets clear rested largely with the householders themselves. An order of 1662 at Preston instructed the inhabitants to sweep and clear the streets in front of their houses and to 'carry away dirt or dung into their backsides, or any other convenient place out of the streets'. While this could have produced clean streets, it may merely have shifted the problem of accumulated rubbish elsewhere within the town.[44] There seems to have been attempts to enforce such orders more rigorously when plague threatened, although at other times their implementation was difficult.

Hugh Peter, the influential Independent preacher and a chaplain of the New Model Army, complained in 1651 of the 'most beastly durtie streets' in London, which caused shoes and clothes to be fouled and made it impossible to keep the interiors of houses clean. He had returned during the early 1640s from a period of exile in Holland, and clearly set his standards of cleanliness by those he had seen in Amsterdam. An Act of Parliament of 1662 that was concerned with the improvement of highways in and around London described them as being 'miry and foul', and so 'very noisom dangerous and inconvenient to the inhabitants'.[45] When James Howel described the state of London in the 1650s he pointed out that the duties of the City's officers included keeping a check on whether any livestock were being kept 'that may cause unwholesomness' and if 'Stable dung, or such kind of noysome filth' was being deposited in the streets and lanes. Yet when he came to consider London's cleanliness, he did so only in relative terms, by comparing it with the state of other European cities, such as Paris, 'the dirt and crott' of which 'may be smelt ten miles off'.[46]

Many provincial towns also had problems with keeping the public places clean. At Bath in 1633 householders were warned against sweeping their rubbish into

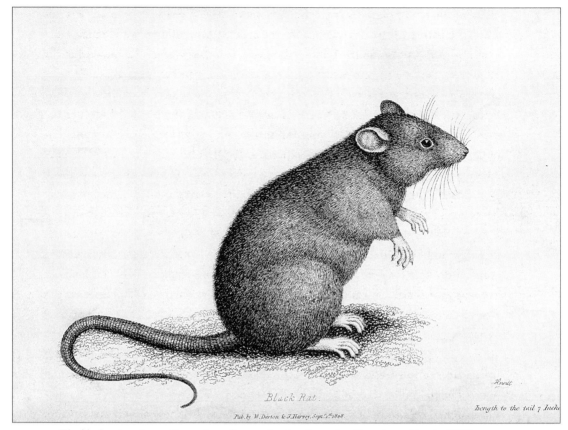

The black rat, rattus rattus, *whose flea carries the plague bacillus. An etching by William Samuel Howitt.* (© The Wellcome Institute Library, London)

the channel that ran down the centre of the street. John Wood was to describe the streets there at the turn of the century as 'like so many dunghills, slaughter houses, pig sties' that contained so much rubbish that pigs were turned loose in them during the day to scavenge.[47] But some places gave a more favourable impression than did London or Bath. Banning carts from the city centre and insisting on the use of sleds instead, as was done at Bristol and Southampton, reduced the problem of horse manure. Towards the end of the seventeenth century Celia Fiennes found the streets at Southampton 'clean swept' and she commented that at Norwich they were 'very clean'.[48]

In one respect Mayerne came close to an important breakthrough in plague control with his recommendation that rodents be killed. Others had noticed that rats emerged from their holes during an outbreak of plague, but they failed to connect their observations with the reasons for the spread of the disease. Only when the nature of the disease and the means of transmission were identified as a result of work by Alexandre Yersin, Shibasaburo Kitasato and P.L. Simond in the 1890s was the role of rats established.[49] The plague bacillus, *Pasteurella Pestis*, is spread by the bite of a rat's flea, *Xenopsylla Cheopis*, which is a parasite of the black rat, *rattus rattus*. The flea feeds on the blood of its infected host and the ingested bacilli multiply to such an extent that they block the proventriculus, the organ at the entrance to the flea's stomach. If the flea transfers from its rat host to a human one and attempts to feed, the passage of the blood into the flea's stomach is obstructed by the blocked proventriculus and so is regurgitated, carrying with it the plague bacilli to the human host.[50] Thus, if action had been taken to implement Mayerne's recommendation that the rat population be systematically killed, much would have been achieved in the control of plague, but the connection between the disease and the rat was not made. Nor was there any awareness of the significance of the observation by Father Antero Maria da San Bonaventura who, during the epidemic in 1657, noted that the pest-house at Genoa was infested by fleas, but that wearing a long waxed robe with a smooth surface gave protection from them. Such robes had come into use in France during the early seventeenth century and had become popular with the plague-doctors in Italy. The development of such effective protection for the doctors was not matched by advances in the treatments for the sick. These largely consisted of the traditional ones of phlebotomy, emetics, blisters and the application of preparations used for treating poisons.[51]

Even though the link with plague was not understood, rats were killed, by poisons or the more direct methods implied by the 'great ratt trapp' that the Charterhouse acquired in 1639. The employment of professional rat-catchers suggests some concern to control the rodent population.[52] Many of the formal regulations, too, were beneficial, especially the isolation in a pest-house of those suspected to have contracted the disease, and of the quarantining of shipping. Yet when they failed, as they did even in the well-administered Italian cities, the other measures were inadequate to prevent an epidemic. Many of the regulations were, in any case, difficult to enforce. This was especially the case with attempts to confine the sick and suspects to their houses. For those who had not contracted the disease, or showed none of the symptoms, being immured with the sick was almost a sentence of death, given the contagiousness of the plague and the high mortality rate. Everyone in isolation faced the risk that if the provisions supplied were inadequate, as often was the case, they

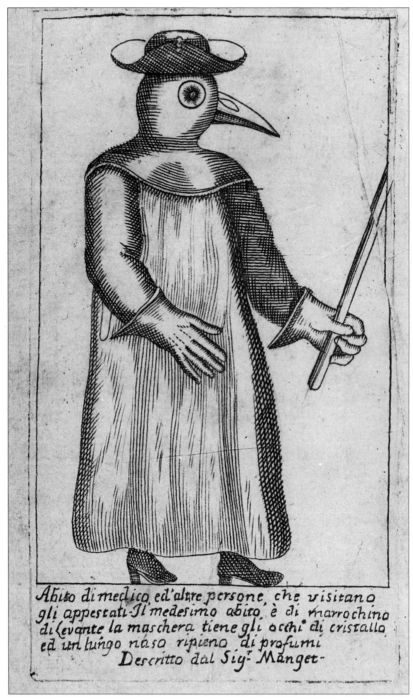

Abito di medico ed'altre persone, che visitano
gli appestati. Il medesimo abito, è di marrochino
di Levante la maschera tiene gli occhi di cristallo
ed un lungo naso ripieno di profumi
      Descritto dal Sig:. Manget-

The long waxed gown and beaked hood covered the whole of the body and offered protection for those treating plague victims. A line engraving after Jean-Jacques Manget. (© The Wellcome Institute Library, London)

would starve, and so they were bound to attempt to come out and try to find food, and perhaps escape. In all respects, being shut up was best avoided, hence the attempts to conceal the symptoms from the searchers, who were not medical staff, or suborn them into giving a false diagnosis. If that failed and the house was marked as one with plague, the distinguishing marks could be removed. In 1630 the Privy Council raised these points in a letter to the Lord Mayor, objecting to the choice of searchers, their concealment of plague cases, failure to seal houses quickly enough when plague was suspected, and negligence in not marking such houses and then ensuring that the marks were not taken away. The vigilance of the watchmen and the inadequate supervision of them were also criticised.[53]

Communities were aware that there was a collective advantage in concealing a possible outbreak, to avoid plague deaths being recorded in the *Bills of Mortality* or the news being spread by other means, which could do tremendous damage. The *Bills* were anxiously consulted by those watching the progress of the disease, both in their own community and in others, where they had interests or perhaps needed to visit. A merchant in Dorchester followed the flare-up of plague at London in 1630 and from the information provided by the *Bills* was able to note in his diary that the greatest number of deaths in a week from the disease had been seventy-seven. Such ready availability of specific information was in itself a cause for the concealment of an outbreak, because potential visitors, suppliers and traders could check the figures and naturally would be deterred once they knew that the disease was increasing.[54] In 1631 as many as 85 per cent of the population of Preston were said to be in need of poor relief, because of their isolation during an outbreak of plague. Faced with disruption on such a scale, concealment was an attractive option that offered the possibility of avoiding social problems and considerable expense. It was made easier if the leading citizens, both magistrates and clergy, left the town to avoid catching the disease themselves. This was something that contemporaries believed that morally they should not do, and the moral argument was reinforced by directions from the Privy Council. Yet, while some remained and conscientiously, and courageously, carried out the duties expected of them in such a crisis, others took evasive action and moved away for their own safety, leaving the implementation of the regulations to the junior officers.[55]

For whatever reason, cases of plague were often kept quiet, not only by the poor, who were afraid that they would be inadequately provided for, but also by the more prominent citizens, and even by the magistrates themselves. In 1604 a

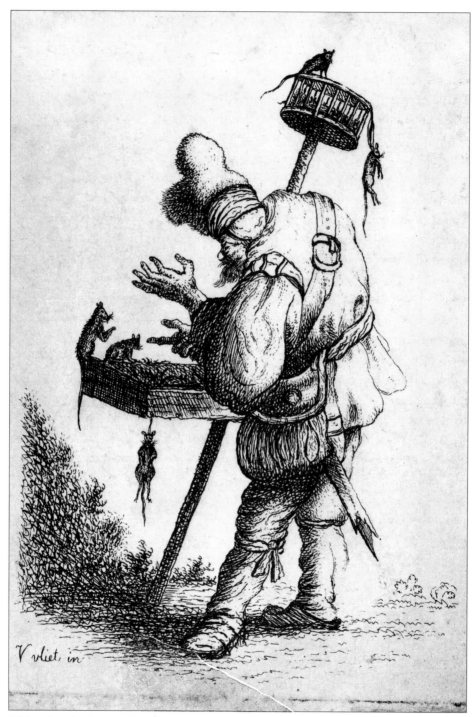

This etching by Jan van der Vliet *shows a* **rat-catcher** *enticing rats into a tray, from which they are transferred to the cage on a pole.* (© The Wellcome Institute Library, London)

servant of John Taylor, an alderman of Gloucester, died of plague, but Taylor concealed the fact. Then another of his servants contracted the disease and Taylor not only once again kept the matter a secret, other than calling in 'a woman experienced therin' to treat the victim, but even permitted the sickly servant to attend the mayor and 'other choise men of the said Cittie' who were being entertained by him. Others then fell ill with the disease and when the truth was discovered Taylor was removed from office and fined £100, his fellow aldermen presumably being outraged that he had so blatantly disregarded the regulations and had put them directly at risk in doing so. Even then, when Taylor's house was quarantined and boarded up his son broke down the boards and threatened to shoot anyone who attempted to keep it sealed. He, too, was fined, and spent an undignified spell in the stocks.[56]

On the other hand, the authorities in some towns were very aware of their responsibilities and erred on the side of caution. At Dorchester, in December 1626, a house was shut up in case the three deaths that had occurred there within fifteen days had been caused by plague, before it was accepted that 'some pestientiall feaver' probably was responsible. In a year when there had been outbreaks of plague at Blandford Forum, Bridport and perhaps Weymouth, coupled with a fear that travellers from northern France might bring the disease, the magistrates at Dorchester clearly felt that their town was under greater threat than usual.[57]

Despite the efforts of magistrates such as those in Dorchester, major outbreaks of plague erupted from time to time throughout the early seventeenth century. The powerlessness even of those who were careful to take precautions against the plague may have engendered a sense of helplessness and encouraged the propensity to ascribe the disasters to the Divinity. Indeed, although the government pressed for the implementation of the regulations, royal proclamations continued to attribute epidemics to God and to call for prayer and fasting to divert His wrath. The outbreak of 1625 was credited to 'the immediate hand of God for the sinnes of this Land, to so visite and correct his people' and its waning in London to His 'infinite goodnesse'.[58] Services on fast days brought people together, however, and thereby risked increasing the spread of the disease. They also provided an opportunity for displays of puritan fervour and so were disliked by the government of Charles I, which ordered that the sermons should be omitted. There was a reaction against this during the puritan ascendancy in the 1640s and 1650s, with providential interpretations of the causes of plague and both local and national fasts observed to try to stem its progress. But, as before,

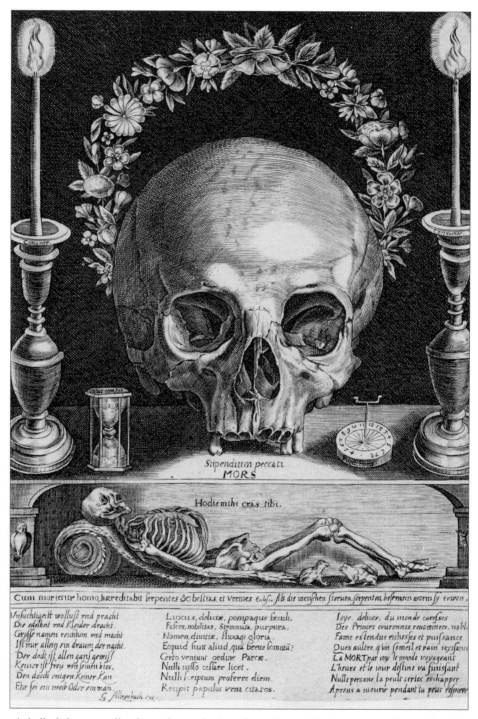

A skull, skeleton, candles, hour-glass and other tokens of mortality, in an engraving attributed to Altzenbach. (© The Wellcome Institute Library, London)

this did not produce a fatalistic resignation to the seemingly inevitable, and practical measures continued to be taken, including the quarantining of shipping from the continent.[59]

Between 1536 and 1670 a plague epidemic struck western Europe on average once every fifteen years. At least two million people died of the disease in France during the first seventy years of the seventeenth century, 35,000 of them at Lyon in the great plague of 1629–32. There were terrible outbreaks in northern and central Italy in the early 1630s, including the *peste di Milano*, which had a devastating effect on Lombardy's population. Florence, Modena and Lucca all suffered high mortality, roughly a third of Venice's inhabitants died of plague during the decade, and a similar proportion of the Tuscan community of Pescia died in an epidemic in 1631. Plague erupted in Germany and the Low Countries in 1623–4 and 1634–5, and in many of the Spanish cities in 1647–50, with particularly severe outbreaks in 1649 at Seville – where half the population was said to have died or fled – and Madrid. In Denmark the effect of epidemics and harvest failures in 1647–51 was to reduce the population by 20 per cent. Even in those Italian states which were recognised to have probably the most complete preventive measures in Europe, there was further high mortality from plague during the mid-1650s. In 1656–7 Rome, Naples and Genoa suffered severely, with more than half the population of Genoa falling victim to the disease.[60]

Knowledge of the occurrence of plague across the continent was readily available from the reports of diplomats, the narratives of travellers, and the correspondence of merchants and their agents. Governments needed information on plague for the influence which it may have on the conduct of diplomacy, the progress of a war, or its impact on trade and the economy, and their diplomats supplied it. It was also as well to have timely warning of an outbreak in another state so that restrictions could be imposed on travellers and goods coming from there. When there was an upsurge of plague in London in 1641 the Venetian envoy notified the *Sopra Proveditori* and the *Proveditori alla Sanita* in Venice, 'so that they may take steps to safeguard the public health'.[61] Travellers necessarily followed a route that would avoid their being quarantined and, for their own safety, places where plague had been reported. In 1637 Richard D'Ewes made his way from Paris to Lyon and lingered there hoping that the plague in Savoy would die down so that he could cross the Alps, but in fact it began to spread towards Lyon, which sent him scurrying to Marseille before finishing his journey to Italy by sea. In 1657 John Reresby waited in vain for the epidemic that affected much of Italy to die down, and eventually curtailed his tour, having seen little more than Venice and Florence. Travellers not only avoided places of their own volition, but also because they were likely to be made most unwelcome if they had come from an area where an outbreak was suspected. Sir Dudley Carleton's entourage travelled through the Tirol and Bavaria mainly at night and were forced to bypass most settlements, crossing fields to avoid them, because they were 'not suffered to pass through any towne nor so much as a village'.[62]

Merchants faced the risk of having their agents quarantined or their goods impounded if they were trading with a place where plague precautions were in force. Hence they were eager for news about the dangers and often were sent reassuring messages by their contacts in a town or city where the disease had been reported. When a Newcastle merchant enquired in 1661 about the plague in Hamburg, he was assured that 'The sickness, blessed be God, is not great, the number last week was but twenty-three, as I read.' Robert Oursel, writing from Rouen in 1668, also adopted a reassuring tone, feeling that the extent of the outbreak of plague there had been exaggerated, yet admitting that already it had claimed forty-one victims. But his attitude was not shared by the authorities of nearby towns, who placed Rouen under quarantine, disrupting its trade during the second half of the year.[63]

The 1630s were an especially difficult period, with Europe experiencing the highest incidence of plague of any decade in the sixteenth and seventeenth centuries. An epidemic in London in 1636 saw the burial of 10,400 plague victims between early April and the middle of December. The contagion spread across much of the country in the following years, affecting both urban and rural communities. Worcester's highest mortality for at least a hundred years came in 1637 and the disease affected country parishes throughout Essex in 1637–40.[64]

The outbreaks continued into the 1640s and were greatly exacerbated by the civil wars in the 1640s, particularly in those towns whose populations were swollen by refugees from the countryside, seeking security, and garrisons of soldiers. In the over-crowded conditions, epidemic disease was a major risk, and many places suffered eruptions of plague or typhus during the war years. Bristol was in the throes of a severe outbreak in September 1645, when it was captured by the New Model Army, and between the autumn of 1644 and that of the following year roughly a quarter of the city's population died, mostly of plague. An outbreak of plague at Oxford, the King's headquarters, in the summer of 1644 saw a range of precautions imposed by the royalist authorities, including quarantining, the opening of the city's pest-house and the building of cabins to

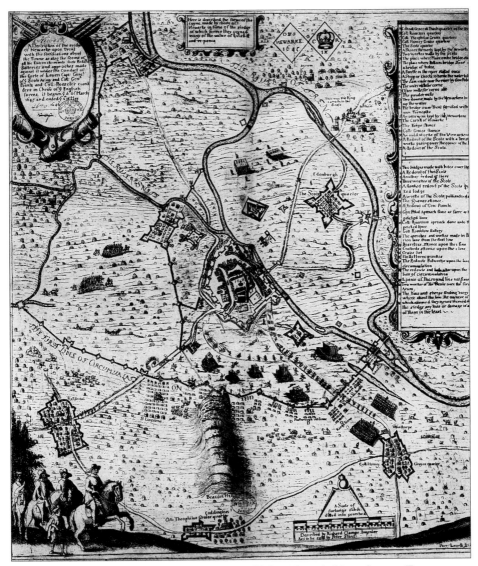

Sieges produced conditions in which the plague could flourish, as in Newark-upon-Trent between 1645 and 1646. (© Crown copyright, NMR)

supplement its accommodation, the killing of cats and dogs, a special tax for relief of the victims and printed *Bills of Mortality*.[65] At Newark guards were posted outside the houses of plague sufferers, but that was not enough to prevent the disease from spreading. By 1646 it was described as 'a miserable stinking infected town' and the epidemic claimed 1,000 victims.[66]

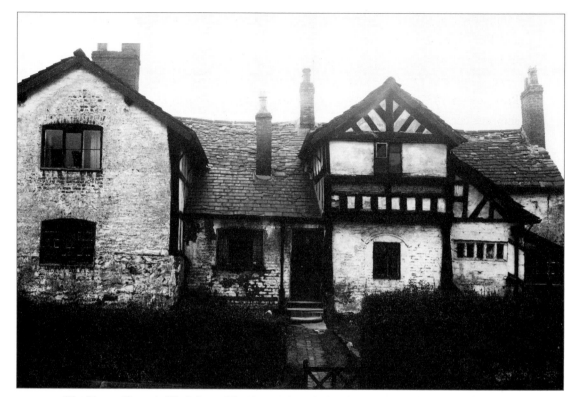

The Plague House in Wash Lane, Warrington, inscribed with the words 'God's providence is mine inheritance' and the date 1652, is said to have been erected to commemorate the owner's escape from the plague. The building has since been demolished. (© Crown copyright, NMR)

Plague struck even unfortified country towns and rural parishes. Warwick closed its gates to the citizens of Stratford-upon-Avon in 1645 because of the plague there, which was serious enough for pest-houses to be built and a rate levied to help maintain the 'poore infected people'. Somerset experienced a plague epidemic in 1645 which spread to Devon in 1646, with over a quarter of the population of the parish of Pilton near Barnstaple recorded as 'dying in the plague and pestilence' during the year.[67]

The outbreaks continued beyond the end of the first Civil War, claiming 3,597 plague deaths in London in 1647 and more than 2,000 at Chester in 1647–8,[68] but they declined in the early 1650s, and between the middle of the decade and the mid-1660s there were no serious outbreaks. Despite the major epidemics in parts of western Europe, including the United Provinces, England and Wales escaped largely unscathed. London's recorded plague deaths averaged fewer than fourteen per annum between 1650 and 1664, compared with 1,500 a year between 1629 and 1636, and 1,072 annually during the late 1640s. This may have led to some complacency, a feeling that the precautions implemented when danger of an epidemic threatened were sufficient to protect the British Isles. During the plague in the United Provinces in 1655 the Protectorate government imposed a period of quarantine on shipping coming from the Dutch ports, and the disease did not spread to Britain.[69]

As the threat diminished, the precautionary measures against plague were gradually relaxed. Norwich discontinued its *Bills of Mortality*, for example. Those for London were still compiled, however, and their potential for purposes other than giving warning of the beginnings of an epidemic was brilliantly shown by John Graunt in his *Natural and Political Observations . . . upon the Bills of Mortality*, published in 1662.[70] A few years before, James Howel had realised their usefulness in estimating the relative sizes of populations of cities, such as London and Amsterdam,[71] but Graunt brought a much wider vision and degree of sophistication to bear, analysing the figures from the previous sixty years to display a range of characteristics of London's population. Comparative data from provincial parishes and outbreaks of plague in continental towns were also considered. Graunt's study included London's plague epidemics since 1592, concluding that 1603 had been 'the greatest Plague year of this Age'. He noticed that high mortality from the disease continued for eight years after the plague of 1603 and twelve years after that of 1636, but that 1625 had been neither preceded or succeeded by high mortality from plague. He implied that a high number of deaths from other diseases, such as 'purple fevers' and smallpox, may indicate an imminent outbreak of plague, citing the figures for the early 1620s. Graunt also studied the seasonality of the disease, remarking that during an epidemic the numbers of deaths could increase and decrease sharply, with a rise from 118 in one week to 993 in the next. His conclusion from this and other evidence in the *Bills* was that 'the Contagion of the Plague depends more upon the Disposition of the Air, than upon the effluvia from the Bodies of men'.[72]

Graunt's explanation of the cause of plague came no nearer to an understanding of the disease than those advanced in Florence more than three hundred years earlier and, despite the preventive measures that had been widely adopted, it still struck with dreadful frequency, killing large numbers. The social pattern of the mortality observed by Boccaccio held good in seventeenth-century England; while the wealthy were able to survive by moving away from the affected areas, the poorer citizens who were not able to leave were the most numerous victims. By the seventeenth century not only the social, but also the geographical and seasonal patterns of plague mortality had been identified, with a general awareness that towns were more severely affected than the countryside and that the most dangerous time was from late spring to early winter. Such knowledge allowed those who could be flexible to take evasive action, limiting the impact of the disease. Even so, none of the administrative measures devised since the Black Death had proved to be successful in preventing an outbreak, and the scale of the mortality during epidemics remained high.

CHAPTER 2

The Great Plague in London

And I will smite the inhabitants of this city, both man and beast: they shall die of a great pestilence.

Jeremiah, 21:6

And in this yeare 1665 and the begining of the yeare following, was there a great Plague in the Cittie and suburbs of London, whereof there dyed for severall weekes together above 8,000 a week, the like whereof was never known in London before.

D.J.H. Clifford (ed.), *The Diaries of Lady Anne Clifford*, p. 177

By the mid-1660s England and Wales had been largely free from plague for ten years, but that was well short of the twenty years that was regarded as the normal interval between outbreaks, and so there should have been little sense of complacency. Any tendency for a relaxation of vigilance ought to have been arrested by news of plague epidemics on the continent. Indeed, attention focused on Turkey, where plague erupted in 1661. This was thought to be the source of the epidemic that began in the Netherlands in 1663 and proved to be one of the worst of the century, with 35,000 deaths in Amsterdam in 1663–4. The outbreak was not confined to the larger cities and towns, but spread out into the countryside, bringing death to small villages.[1] Not only was this epidemic much closer to the British Isles than those which had affected southern Europe in the 1650s, but the United Provinces was a major trading partner and so there was a considerable danger that the disease would spread to English ports.

The Privy Council responded to the risk by imposing controls on shipping, with a period of quarantine for vessels coming from ports where plague had been present.[2] Only five recorded deaths from the disease occurred in London during 1664, and there was no hint of the epidemic to come.

Conditions in the early months of the following year were, according to John Gadbury, not conducive to plague.[3] The winter was a comparatively severe one, with frosts beginning in December and continuing into March. Average monthly temperatures in the Midlands were no higher than 1°C during January and February, and London experienced similar cold weather. Both John Evelyn and Samuel Pepys noted that it was very cold towards the end of December and Pepys described 6 February as one of the coldest days ever experienced in England. The frost was so prolonged and intense that the Thames at London was frozen over for two consecutive months. At the end of March Pepys remarked that it had been 'as hard a winter as any hath been these many years' and Simon Patrick, rector of St Paul's, Covent Garden, wrote that the hard frost continued until almost the middle of April. Memories of weather conditions tend to be unreliable, with the most recent seasons seeming to be extreme. In fact, the winter of 1662/3 had produced equally low average temperatures in the Midlands, and that of 1657/8 had also been a harsh one.[4]

Even in the cold winter weather, some suspected cases of plague occurred, but the victims recovered. Yet the spring weather did not bring a sharp upsurge of cases, despite Nathaniel Hodges's comment that 'upon the frost breaking, the contagion got ground'.[5] Only three fatalities from plague were recorded in the *Bills of Mortality* before the end of April, and forty-three more during May.[6] But while the numbers returned for May were fewer than 3 per cent of all deaths notified during the month, already there was cause for concern. The Earl of Clarendon, the Lord Chancellor, later recalled that although plague cases had been reported so far 'only in the outskirts of the town and in the most obscure alleys, amongst the poorest people', those who remembered the way in which the epidemic of 1625 had begun 'foretold a fearful summer'. By 28 May Lady Sandwich was so 'afeared of the sickness' that she decided to leave London, and in *The Intelligencer* for 5 June, Roger L'Estrange, Surveyor of the Press, felt the need to try to quash the rumours that 'multitudes' were dying every week of the disease, by giving the actual numbers of plague dead as recorded in the *Bills*.[7]

Despite L'Estrange's efforts, the common attitude was to place no great reliance upon those figures, which did indeed under-record the true numbers, because of concealment of the cause of death. For example, two plague deaths were entered in the burial register of St Paul's, Covent Garden during these months, but they were not included in the *Bills*, and towards the end of May John Allin, living in Horsleydown on the south bank downstream from Southwark, wrote that it was thought that deaths from the disease were three times the recorded number.[8] The information in the *Bills* continued to be treated with scepticism as an official version that under-stated the figures. In the middle

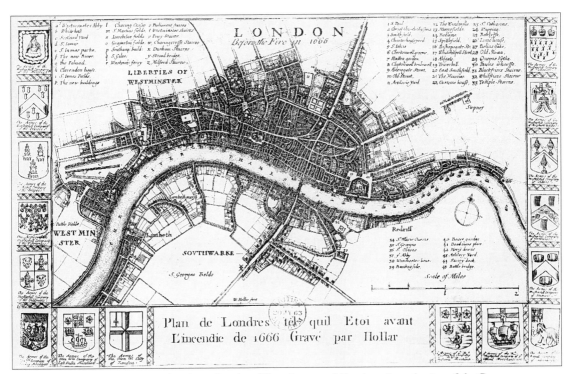

Wenceslaus Hollar's plan shows London, Westminster and Southwark at the tine of the Great Plague. (© Crown copyright, NMR)

of June the Venetian ambassador declared that, as 112 plague deaths were admitted to in one week, the true number could be twice as many, and his estimate of the attributed and actual statistics for deaths from the disease in the third week of July suggests a disparity of more than 40 per cent.[9] While his evaluation could not have had a secure basis, the widening gap between the total deaths and those categorised as being from plague was in itself likely to arouse suspicion, if only because the numbers of non-plague deaths were so much higher than in a normal year.

The motives for minimising the scale of the outbreak included the need to curb the growing concern, and so prevent the premature departure of those who were inclined to leave, and the impact upon the diplomatic situation, for an epidemic would be interpreted as a source of weakness that could impair the country's ability to continue to wage the war against the Dutch, which had broken out in March. News of an outbreak of plague could also injure overseas trade, as other countries banned ships from England entering their ports. The figures from the

Bills were available on the continent soon after they had been released.[10] Yet scepticism about the returns continued even when the scale and nature of the disaster could no longer be concealed. Indeed, inaccurate totals were an accumulation of false returns from individual households and the parish clerks, and need not be attributed entirely to official adjustments when a *Bill* was being compiled. As in earlier epidemics, the searchers would be urged by the victims' families to conceal the cause of death, to avoid the shutting up of houses. John Graunt characterised searchers as inebriates who were open to bribery to falsify the cause. Furthermore, the parish officers were aware of the effects on their district of a high return of plague deaths, in terms of residents moving away and visitors or passers-by avoiding the area, with the problems that ensued. Thus, for the last week of August the parish clerk of St Olave's, Hart Street returned a total of nine deaths, six of them from plague, and these were the figures in the *Bill*, although he admitted that all had been from plague.[11]

Whatever the inaccuracies in the returns, they indicate that the situation steadily worsened during June. Those for its first week show that fewer than 10 per cent of the 405 reported deaths were caused by plague, but by the final week the proportion had risen to 40 per cent and the total to 684. The number of deaths across the capital had been running above the average of the previous ten years for most of the year and from the third week of June were more than twice the average. Sir William Petty's rule of thumb was that when there were 100 deaths in a week 'the Plague is begun'.[12] This level was reached in the middle of the month, by which time a migration out of London was under way. In a letter written on 13 June it was reported that all the gentry had either left London or were preparing to leave, and that the king and queen were to go to Hampton Court the following week.[13]

Yet by no means everyone had taken alarm or felt the need either to move out of London or take care to limit their social contacts. Thomas Rugg noted in May that the theatres were 'thronged with people of all sorts and sizes' and he was reassured by the fact that the figures for the month showed that plague deaths had occurred in only 5 of the 130 parishes recorded in the *Bills*.[14] Sir Thomas Viner, a goldsmith and former Lord Mayor, died on 11 May and, as was customary for someone of his standing, there was a delay before his funeral, so that suitable arrangements could be made. The service was held at the church of St Mary Woolnoth on 1 June and was a grand affair that drew a large number of people. The Lord Mayor and aldermen attended, as did the boys and pensioners of Christ's Hospital. The funeral gathering was held at the halls of the

Goldsmiths' and Haberdashers' companies, and both were full of people, with 'the number of the company very great'.[15] It was a common practice to forbid gatherings on such a scale during an epidemic, but the corporation clearly thought that such precautions were not yet necessary within the City.

John Evelyn spent much of the first half of June in Kent and the remainder at his house at Wotton in Surrey, with several visits to London and the court. His first mention of the plague in his diary was on 28 June, in respect of the meetings of the Royal Society coming to an end earlier in the summer than was usual, because of the risk. Yet he must have been aware of the growing danger, and a month earlier he had noted that the curate at Wotton had preached on Psalm 91, with its assurance of God's protection in perilous times, including those of the noisome pestilence and the plague. Despite his awareness of the developing outbreak, the diary entries do not suggest that he felt threatened by it.[16]

A part of the reason for the lack of immediate concern both in the City and at Whitehall may have been the localisation of the plague deaths. In its early stages the outbreak was centred in St Giles-in-the-Fields, a comparatively large parish of 1,500 households almost on the edge of the built-up area to the west of the City, where suspected cases had been noted towards the end of 1664. Steps were taken to close houses where victims had been identified and a pest-house for the parish was built at Marylebone. Nevertheless, St Giles continued to be the worst afflicted area, with 343 burials of plague victims during June, out of the total of 590 recorded in the *Bills*.[17]

In an attempt to isolate the plague there, on 21 June the Privy Council directed the officers of the adjoining parishes to set warders on the streets and other passageways from St Giles, to stop those suspected of coming from infected houses or districts, as well as vagrants and other 'loose persons'.[18] This policy may have been difficult to implement and perhaps was adopted rather too late, for a growing number of cases were reported in the neighbouring districts. On 7 June Pepys noticed houses in Drury Lane marked with the regulation red cross and the inscription 'Lord have mercy upon us', and ten days later had, as he imagined, his first brush with danger when the driver of the coach in which he was travelling along Holborn gradually brought the vehicle to a halt and alighted, telling his passenger that he was 'suddenly stroke very sick and almost blind'.[19] But other areas, well away from St Giles, also began to record plague deaths. The disease had penetrated into the City during the first week of May and in early June deaths from plague were recorded in Fenchurch Street and Broad Street, as well as in the extramural parishes of St Botolph, Bishopsgate, and St Mary, Whitechapel, east of the City. While it is possible that either those fleeing from the outbreak in and around St Giles, or others who were still trying to continue with their normal routines, may have spread the infection to the other districts, it is also conceivable that there were several sources of infection. This was the opinion of the apothecary William Boghurst, who wrote that the plague 'fell upon severall places of this City and Suburbs like raine'.[20] It was not only the number of cases recorded in the *Bills*, but also the increasing area affected, upon which individuals based their assessment of the scale of the danger and which produced the rising tide of anxiety and departures from London of those who were able to leave.

While the spread of the plague could be charted from the *Bills*, its origins were uncertain. England's relative freedom from the disease over the previous few years suggested that such a large-scale epidemic had resulted from infection brought from abroad, with the Netherlands regarded as the likely source. Nathaniel Hodges was both specific, in attributing the outbreak to cloth brought from the Levant through Amsterdam to London, and undecided, describing it as 'a small spark, from an unknown cause'. A source of infection among imported goods or travellers coming from the continent would suggest an initial outbreak in the riverside parishes. In fact, the area around St Giles, well away from the Thames wharves, was recognised as the centre of the outbreak, although notice of an early plague death in 1665 was returned from the riverside parish of St Mary Savoy.[21]

Contemporaries also linked the eruption in 1665 to the weather. Pepys noted that it was hot in the middle of May and in early June referred to 'the mighty heat of the weather'. He described 7 June as the hottest day he had ever experienced and the warmest day at that time of the year that anyone could remember. The Venetian ambassador also mentioned the 'intense heat' and the fear that the plague would greatly increase as a result.[22] But the temperature figures for the Midlands do not support the impression of an unusually warm spring and summer, and Hodges described the summer in London as being not too hot and with fresh breezes, in other words not the conditions that would produce the stagnant and corrupted air which contemporaries regarded as conducive to the spread of plague.[23] A more distinctive feature of the spring and early summer was its unusual dryness. Boghurst noted that the plague 'was ushered in' with seven months of dry weather and westerly winds. He recalled that little or no rain fell during that period, except for a few showers towards the end of April. This resulted in a poor hay crop, which was also commented on by Richard Baxter, at Acton, who thought that only four loads were harvested where forty would have been taken in a normal year. Baxter wrote that the winter, spring and summer were together the driest in living memory. This is supported by Pepys, who noted that the rain in late April was very welcome and settled the dust, and made few further notes of rainfall before the end of June.[24]

During June plague cases became more common in Westminster, even close to Whitehall Palace, where several people died in just one alley.[25] In the early part of the month the attention of the court was focused rather on the fleet's successful engagement with the Dutch at the battle of Lowestoft on 3 June, and then the return of the Duke of York and the other naval commanders. It would not have been tactful to have withdrawn from court before having offered congratulations to the proud victors, who did not arrive at Whitehall until 16 June. But thereafter

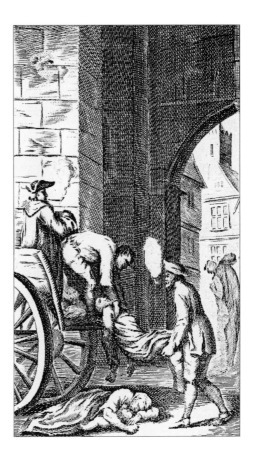

Samuel Wale's mid-eighteenth-century drawing shows victims of the plague in 1665 being lifted into the dead cart. Smoking was thought to offer protection against the plague. (© The Wellcome Institute Library, London)

the threat of the plague produced a gradual stream of departures, including the Earl of Southampton, the Lord Treasurer, who had left by 17 June, until the whole court moved out of Whitehall at the end of the month, going first to Syon House and then, on 9 July, to Hampton Court. The king accompanied his mother, Henrietta Maria, to Dover on her way to France. By the end of June Pepys found that only the Duke of Albemarle, the Earl of Clarendon and Sir Henry Bennet among the 'great statesmen' were left in the capital, although other leading figures were also to remain during the epidemic, including the Earl of Craven, the Archbishop of Canterbury, the Bishop of London and Sir John Lawrence, the Lord Mayor. According to the Venetian ambassador, Lawrence had a glass case made for himself, from within which he supervised business and received visitors.[26]

On 5 June the theatres were closed on the orders of the Lord Chamberlain. The Inns of Court broke up around the middle of the month. At Lincoln's Inn rules were put in place for the regulation of the Inn during the remainder of the plague, which involved control of visitors and a strict overnight curfew on everyone from ten o'clock until morning. In early July the Lord Mayor ordered that all schools in the City were to close until the end of September. The scholars of Westminster School also departed; Dr Busby, the headmaster, took them to Chiswick, but, when that proved to be unsafe, told them that they were free to return to their own homes.[27]

While the plague had caused much disruption around Westminster, the City was still relatively free from the disease, with just eighteen plague deaths recorded within the walls in the four weeks to 27 June. Yet on the 21st Pepys, at Cripplegate, found 'all the town almost going out of town, the coaches and waggons being all full of people going into the country'.[28] But this was still a gradual process, for not everyone was panicked into leaving and on 18 July Samuel Herne wrote to his tutor at Clare Hall, Cambridge that 'there is but very little notice tooke of the sicknesse here in London', except that St Giles was to be avoided. Elsewhere in his letter, however, he rather contradicted this impression, mentioning that 'the citizens begin to shut up apace' and that there were few houses still open even in the Strand and at the Royal Exchange in Cornhill.[29] Herne's account mixed an attempt at reassurance with an awareness of the scale of the growing crisis.

The *Bills* for the week in which Herne wrote show that plague deaths in the parishes within the walls had doubled to fifty-six since the last set of figures, and were increasing steadily elsewhere. The City parishes outside the walls saw a rise from 166 plague deaths in the first week of July, to 755 in the last week, and the Westminster parishes an increase from 105 to 322 over that period. In the 130 parishes recorded by the *Bills*, the weekly number of deaths from the disease rose from 470 to 2,010 during the month, and total deaths from 1,006 to 3,014. By the end of July the mortality rate was almost ten times that of the preceding ten years, and even in the area within the walls it was four times that level. With 8,828 deaths during July, 5,667 of them from plague, there was no disguising the scale of the unfolding disaster. Nor was there any indication of the beginning of a decline, for recorded deaths at the end of July were three times the number noted for the last week of June and those attributed to plague had increased more than fourfold, while the number of parishes in which deaths from the disease had occurred had risen from thirty-three to seventy-three. The *Bills* gave no cause for hope of an imminent end to the epidemic, and previous outbreaks had shown that the summer months were likely to be the worst of all.

Pepys packed his mother off home to Huntingdonshire on 22 June and his wife and her maids to Woolwich on 5 July. Towards the end of July he began to fear for the safety of his cousin Kate Joyce, because there had been forty deaths in one week in the parish where she and her husband Anthony kept a tallow-chandler's shop. Yet Pepys had to use 'all the vehemence and Rhetorique' he could muster to persuade Anthony that she should leave. He was not keen, presenting 'some simple reasons, but most that of profit' why she should stay, but eventually was induced to agree that she should go to friends at Windsor, and not to Huntingdonshire as Pepys had wanted, because of the distance 'if either of them should be ill'. Like Anthony Joyce, Pepys remained in London for the time being, but from early September he spent his nights at Woolwich, although he continued to go regularly to his house and office in Seething Lane. In contrast, Richard Baxter made a complete break, although he lived well outside the city, at Acton, and so in comparative safety. He left at the end of July, when plague appeared in the parish, and moved to Great Hampden in Buckinghamshire.[30] Such departures, with the tendency of many citizens to go into public places as little as possible, produced a growing air of desertion. Evelyn was struck by the emptiness of the streets, the closed shops and the 'mournefull silence'.[31]

Those who were unable or unwilling to leave could try to avoid infection by taking sensible precautions and limiting their contact with others as much as possible. Henry Oldenburg, the secretary of the Royal Society, had considered that if plague was reported in the row of houses where he lived he would go into the country, but at the end of July he told one of his correspondents that he

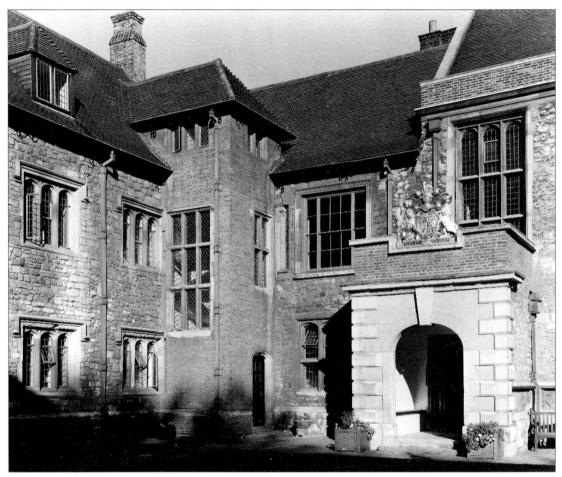

The secluded buildings of the Charterhouse were Edward Swan's refuge throughout the epidemic. (© Crown copyright, NMR)

intended to remain at his house in Pall Mall, endeavouring 'to banish both fear and overconfidence, leading a regular life and avoiding infected places as much as I can'. A month later he reported that very few houses where the occupants lived 'orderly and comfortably' and had healthy constitutions had been infected, whereas those 'wanting necessaries and comfortable relief' suffered most.[32] A degree of selfishness was acceptable. As Edward Wood wrote to his agent John Pack, who lived in Thames Street, 'every man is bound to use the meanes for his preservation in this sad visitation'. He had earlier offered Pack the simple advice to 'goe abroad as litle as may be', while he chose to remain at Littleton, near Staines. Sir Robert Long, too, stayed out of London, telling his clerk to keep his house in New Palace Yard as insulated as possible, not letting anyone out, or permitting visitors to come to either the house or the office. Such isolation was seen to be the safest course. At the end of the following January Edward Swan, one of the pensioners at the Charterhouse on the northern edge of the City, wrote that he had not been out of the almshouse once in the previous seven months.[33]

Oldenburg and Swan can readily be equated with the citizens of Florence who shut themselves away during the Black Death. Another of Boccaccio's categories was represented by Samuel Pepys and Simon Patrick, who were careful, yet continued to go about their business. Pepys was well aware of the progress of the disease, noting the figures in the *Bills* and the districts where it was present. He scrupulously put his affairs in order, sorting his papers, making up his accounts, packing his books into chests, and getting 'all things in the best and speediest order I can'. He also re-drafted his will, conscious that 'a man cannot depend on living two days to an end'. In some respects he was fastidious, not wishing to visit a house two doors away from one which had been shut up, avoiding unnecessary conversations in public places, not attending his parish church for almost five months, and even not wearing his new periwig for a while, because the plague had been in Westminster when he had bought it there. Diet was a consideration, for the safety of daily provisions was questionable, with 'the butcheries being everywhere visited', Pepys's own baker having died of the plague, together with his entire family, and his brewer's house shut up. He noted those occasions when he may have been exposed to the disease, such as when he 'met a dead Corpse, of the plague' in a narrow alley, or passed 'close by the bearers with a dead corpse of the plague', and when he had news of those who lived near to him, or that he may have been in contact with, who had been taken ill or died. On the other hand he quite consciously took unnecessary risks, such as going to Deptford for an amorous encounter in a house where 'round about and next door on every side is the plague', enjoying oysters out of a barrel sent from Colchester, knowing that the town was suffering badly with the disease, and even setting out to Moorfields to try to see a corpse being carried to burial in the plague-pits there.[34]

Despite his awareness of the extent and impact of the disease at both personal and general levels, which engendered gloomy comments from time to time, Pepys was by no means an unhappy man during the outbreak. He occasionally refers to being 'very merry' and one night he had the best dream that he could remember, in which he had Lady Castlemaine in his arms and she allowed him 'all the dalliance I desired'. These were more than occasional moods, for he noted that he ended July 'with the greatest glut of content that ever I had' and as September came to a close he summarised the previous three months in much the same terms, as having been 'much the greatest' that he had ever experienced 'for joy, health and profit'. Nor had his impression changed when he came to look back over the whole year, commenting that 'I have never lived so merrily . . . as I have done this plague-time'.[35]

As a clergyman, Simon Patrick could not be as selective in choosing his company as could Pepys. He had to conduct services and deliver his sermons, administer alms to his parishioners and meet others who may be carrying the disease. The wife and one of the children of his parish clerk died of plague, and a visit to a friend also put him at risk, for the friend was entertaining another clergyman, who died just a few days later. Yet Patrick, too, was essentially cautious, without being too restricted in his movements, going out from time to time and walking to Battersea and back to visit his brother. He was careful to be neither too bold and confident on the one hand, or too timorous on the other, noting that some were struck by the plague 'that stir not half so much abroad as I'. When he bought a pair of stockings, he was sure that the friend from whom he purchased them was clear of the plague, and that the stockings had been in his shop for a long time. Other risks had to be run. He realised that the containers of wine and beer might carry the disease, and bread was thought to be a possible means by which it was transmitted, but he had to buy those items. Yet he did alter his habits to some extent, admitting that 'I have quite changed my Diet. I eat boiled Meats & Broths more than I used: something at Supper also.'[36]

For all his care and change of regime, Patrick did have some scares. His brother was taken ill on one occasion, his servant's face swelled up, and Patrick himself began to suffer with 'a sore pain in my leg . . . which made me suspect some touch of the plague'.[37] As sores or buboes on the leg were indeed symptoms of the disease, Patrick's anxiety was understandable, but in the circumstances the reaction to almost any illness was that it could be the beginnings of the plague. Evelyn's family reacted with alarm when he had a fainting fit, not surprisingly, for he had recently been in places containing plague victims. Some took quite drastic action if they suspected an acquaintance or colleague of being ill. When his clerk Will Hewer came in one day and complained of a headache, one of the early signs of the onset of plague, Pepys was so appalled that he told the servants to 'get him out of the house . . . without discouraging him'. Hewer later went to his lodgings, but the following day was back at work, perfectly recovered from what had been

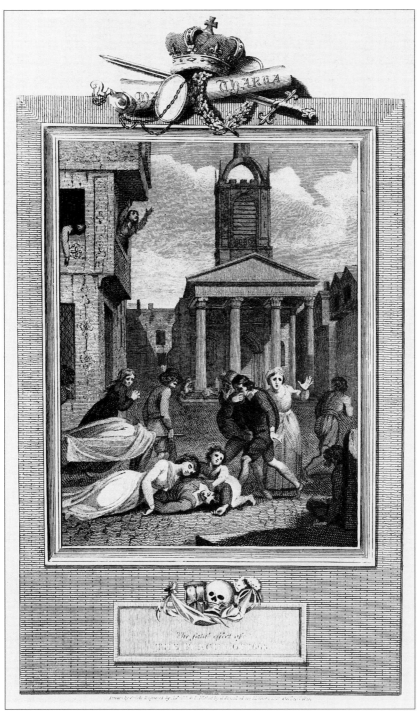

Robert Smirke's impression of a scene in London during the Great Plague, drawn in 1810.
(© Guildhall Library, Corporation of London)

no more than a headache. William Outram, rector of St Mary Woolnoth in the City, was visited by a fellow clergyman, but suspecting from his appearance that he was unwell he instructed his servant that if he returned, he should not let him in. Pepys noted how the epidemic had produced a cruelty in the way that people treated each other.[38]

Those who were ill of another disease were likely to be dealt with as though they were plague victims, or to be left without proper nursing in case their illness was plague. William Taswell wrote that his household was afflicted with the plague and two maidservants were sent to the pest-house. Both of his parents were taken ill and his brother had 'a tumour in his thigh'. None of the family died, however, and Taswell does not specify if their ailments had been plague or not, but nor does he relate whether the servants did indeed have the disease, or their fate. The mortality rate at any pest-house was very high, although some victims did survive.[39] Early in September Patrick saw a group of about thirty people making their way along the Strand carrying white sticks. They were the patients of the doctor at one of the pest-houses who had recovered from the plague and were on their way to the justices, to obtain official certification of their recovery.[40]

In such a climate of anxiety and fear many put their faith in quack medicines and homespun remedies. Thomas Vincent noted that 'without some antidote few stir abroad in the morning'. Sir Walter Raleigh's cordial was very popular and Lady Giffard felt that its use had saved her family from plague during the epidemic.[41] Pepys, in contrast, seemed to take a sceptical view of those which were on offer, observing that some suppliers said one thing and some another, but after noticing houses that were shut up and marked as plague-houses, he had recourse to a plug of tobacco to smell and chew. Tobacco was highly prized as a prophylactic against plague and was one of the more conventional preventive substances on offer. A later tradition held that no London tobacconist died of plague during the epidemic.[42]

The suppliers of nostrums placed advertisements in the newspapers from the middle of May, often citing the success of their potion in previous outbreaks, especially that of 1625. Their cures were priced according to the means of their customers, Henry Eversden offering Sir Theodore de Medde's Anti-pharmocan for just 3d, yet charging 2s 6d for a glass containing five ounces of the Universal Elixir.[43] For the apothecaries who stayed in London, this was potentially a very profitable time. Boghurst saw fifty or sixty patients a day and the Charterhouse's apothecary, William Rawlins, presented a bill for £10 4s 5d for physic supplied there during the epidemic, even though many of the residents had left when the plague began to threaten.[44] Rawlins survived to present his bill for payment, but although supplying medicines was a lucrative business, it was also an exceptionally dangerous one, especially as some apothecaries were prepared to visit the sufferers. Boghurst nursed his patients in their homes, remaining until they died and even staying to help place them in their coffins, while another apothecary described to Simon Patrick, with whom he shared a coach, the plague victims he had visited, detailing 'the nature of their swellings and sores'. By the middle of October, according to Pepys, only one apothecary was still alive in Westminster.[45]

Nathaniel Hodges, a physician, took some satisfaction from the fact that 'these blowers of the pestilential flame' were themselves victims of the epidemic, thus in some way excusing the neglect of the magistrates who had allowed them to continue to peddle their useless medicines. He was severe in his condemnation of those 'chymists and quacks' who were 'equal strangers to all learning as well as physic' and yet 'thrust into every hand some trash or other under the disguise of a pompous title'. Hodges believed that these 'wicked impostors' supplied medicines that were 'more fatal than the plague' and added to the numbers who had died, for 'hardly a person escaped that trusted to their delusions'. Yet a member of his own profession, Dr Tristran Inard, advertised a 'Grand Preservative, or Antidote Epidemical' and, although Hodges regarded sack as the best antidote, he acknowledged that it could be impregnated with wormwood or angelica.[46]

Hodges's uncompromising reaction partly reflected the tension between the physicians and the apothecaries, which produced a pamphlet war that continued for the remainder of the century. The physicians particularly resented those apothecaries who acted independently of them, by attending patients and prescribing treatments. Boghurst justified this with the comment that the apothecaries were 'bound by their undertakings to stay and help' the victims of plague, as they would with those suffering from another disease, and that members of any profession were committed to 'the good and the evil, the pleasure and the pain, the profit and the inconvenience altogether'. In any case, the distinction which the College of Physicians sought to maintain between the three branches of the medical profession – the physicians, surgeons and apothecaries – did not exist in practice. Indeed, many apothecaries virtually acted as general practitioners.[47]

Hodges's comments may also have reflected a common mistrust of the efficacy of the apothecaries' remedies, which, with their cost, led many to prepare their own concoctions. John Conyers remained at his shop in Fleet Street throughout the epidemic, and was aware of such criticism, judging from the title of his pamphlet *Direction for the prevention and cure of the plague, fitted for the poorer sort*.[48] This was just one of forty-six publications concerned with plague that appeared in 1665 and 1666, and books issued during earlier outbreaks were also consulted. Robert Boyle wrote from Oxford that he had a copy of a book published in 1605 containing remedies and suggested that it could be reprinted, with the addition of those approved in the plague of 1625.[49] Sir Robert Long advocated taking a small dose of a compound known as London treacle every morning, or the kernel of a walnut with five leaves of rue and a grain of salt, beaten together and roasted in a fig.[50] Treacle was a common nostrum, recommended in a broadsheet distributed by the parish churchwardens, and by the College of Physicians as one of the fillings, with rue and a fig, of a 'greate onion' which, when roasted, should be applied to a plague sore for up to three hours. Simon Patrick told a friend that 'now and then I take a little Treacle' and Pepys took some Venice treacle before he went to bed one evening in July, when he felt 'out of order'.[51] John Allin's favoured protection was to keep a piece of gold in the mouth, preferably a coin of Elizabeth's reign, when walking out or being visited by the sick. He was scornful of the faith which many placed in amulets made of toad poison, considering that a preparation of his own would prove to be an effective remedy. Others took the more drastic and dangerous step of trying to contract syphilis, believing that it conferred immunity from plague. In 1665 eighty-six deaths from the French pox were returned in the *Bills*, compared with fewer than twenty in an average year, although Graunt warned that the disease was always under-recorded, with its victims entered in the category of 'consumption'.[52]

A procedure commonly taken during plague epidemics that was also instituted in 1665 was the control of livestock and domestic animals, and the extermination of stray animals who scavenged. The dog-catcher for St Margaret's, Westminster was paid for burying 353 dog corpses.[53] The City corporation also adopted a policy of regulating domestic animals, by prohibiting the keeping of pigs, dogs, cats, pigeons and rabbits. Stray pigs were to be impounded and dogs killed. The corporation's dog-catcher claimed for payment for 4,380 dogs slaughtered. Sir Robert Long was concerned about the danger posed by rodents and cats, for he told his clerk, 'take all course you can agaynst the ratts, and take care of the catts; the little ones that will not stirre out may be kept, the great ones must be kiled or sent away'.[54]

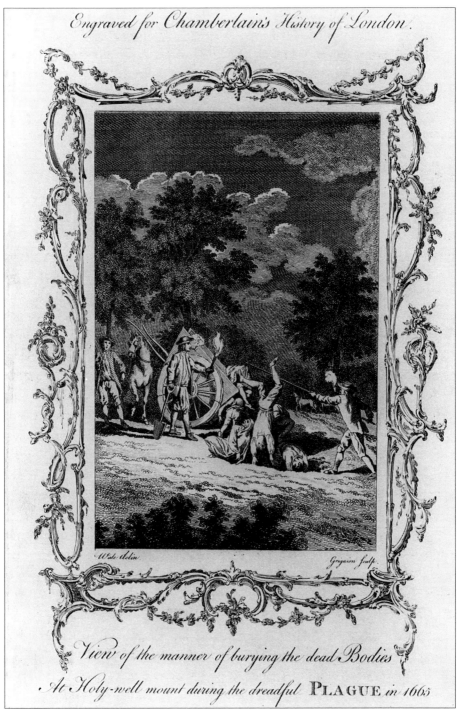

Samuel Wale's depiction of the burial of plague victims at Holywell Lane, Shoreditch during the Great Plague. (© Guildhall Library, Corporation of London)

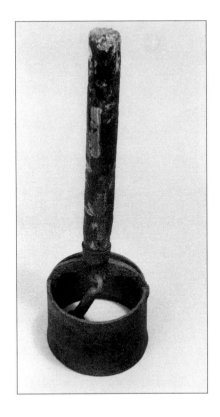

A seventeenth-century plague bell, used to warn of the passing of the dead cart. (© Museum of London)

Fumigation of houses was also a common response, and one which was officially encouraged. Prompted by the Privy Council, the Royal College of Physicians issued its *Necessary Directions* for the prevention and cure of the plague 'with divers remedies of small charge'. Among other recommendations, it advocated the potentially hazardous steps of lighting fires and frequent discharging of guns. It was a measure of the scale of the threat posed by the plague, and the fear that it induced, that such methods should be encouraged, despite the obvious fire risks which they presented during such a dry period. The advice was followed by both the magistrates and individual householders, prompted by the government.[55]

The Privy Council favoured the remedies recommended by James Angier and directed the justices to adopt them. They included a fumigant consisting of a mixture of brimstone, saltpetre and amber. Early in June his methods were tested by the Middlesex justices at a house in Newton Street, off High Holborn, where four occupants had died of the plague and two of the remaining eight were ill with the disease. After Angier's servant had disinfected or fumigated that and other houses, no further deaths were recorded in them. His mixture must have produced a strong and obnoxious stench that all rodents would have found unbearable. In 1670 a warrant was issued for Angier to be paid £86 out of the Exchequer 'for fumes in the late sickness time'.[56] The Lord Mayor ordered that the occupants of houses that had been closed should not be allowed out at the end of the quarantine period until both house and goods had been 'well aired & fumed with brimstone or other knowne good correction of the infeccon'. The post office, in Cloak Lane, Dowgate was fumigated morning and evening, to such an extent that those working there could hardly see each other across the room, and letters were aired over vinegar before being dispatched. Householders, too, regarded fumigation as a preventive measure. Sir Robert Long told his clerk that combustible materials should be gathered and burnt daily, and Dr John Worthington commended the burning of brimstone twice each day to fumigate a house. William Sancroft, Dean of St Paul's, was assured that his London residence was fumigated twice a week, with a rather exotic compound of brimstone, hops, pepper and frankincense.[57]

An extension of the practice of fumigating houses was the lighting of fires in the streets. This had been done in earlier epidemics but was not carried out in 1665 until early September. This may have been because of doubts about the effectiveness of such a strategy, not least among the physicians. Hodges regarded it as a 'showy and expensive' policy that was 'of no effect' because the air in itself was not infected, and Clarendon had already reached the same conclusion. Perhaps by the beginning of September it was thought that anything should be tried that might check the remorseless increase of plague deaths. During the four weeks of August the numbers of deaths attributed to the disease had been 2,817, 3,880, 4,237 and 6,102, with 22,413 deaths from all causes in this period, and the number of parishes in which plague victims had died had risen from 86 to 113. The peak of the epidemic in 1603 had been the last week of August and in that of 1625 the third week, but these dates were passed without any sign of a slackening in the rising death toll. Indeed, the first week of September saw a further increase, to 6,988, which Pepys regarded as 'a most dreadfull Number' and caused Clarendon to despair of an improvement in the figures, writing that if those for the following week also showed an increase he would 'despayre of the whole winter'.[58] It was against this background that the street fires were tried, one to every twelve houses – six on each side of the street – with the watchmen checking that they were kept alight. The bonfires required a considerable expenditure on fuel, including tar barrels, which cost the City parishes between £3 10s and £5 6s.

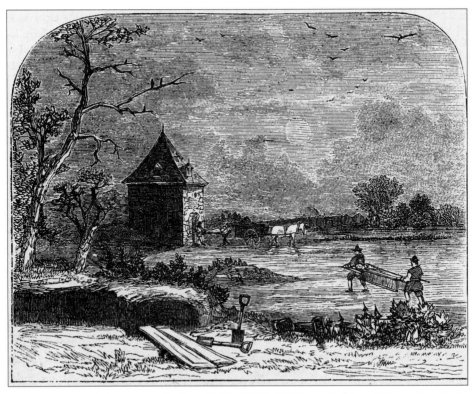

The pest-house and plague pit at Finsbury Fields. (© The Wellcome Institute Library, London)

They burned for three days and nights, until doused by the heavy rain which fell on 9 September, ending a dry spell that had lasted since the middle of August. The drought of the previous winter and spring, and the hot spell early in June, had not been followed by a particularly warm summer, with both July and August somewhat cooler than the average for the previous six years.[59]

Hodges found justification for his scepticism of the policy in the continuing high numbers of plague deaths in the week after the fires, with 6,544 recorded. In fact, this was a decrease of 444, the first since the epidemic had begun, and it engendered a burst of optimism, but in the following week, beginning 12 September, the numbers rose again, to 7,165. This, however, was to prove the peak and the next week saw a fall, to 5,533 deaths from plague. Clarendon was at Oxford with the court, and his relief at the news was obvious, especially as he had received a gloomy forecast from the Archbishop of Canterbury, who was still at Lambeth Palace. When he was given the actual figures, Clarendon replied in a lightly teasing tone, 'I do thanke your Lordship with all my hearte for keepinge us wakinge all this night with the dismall newes of the continuance of the Bill, to the same number as the last week, with only an abatement of 3 of the plague', when in fact the decrease was 1,632 of plague and 1,837 in all.[60] Here at last was a sign that the worst had passed and the epidemic in London was on the decline. The *Bills* recorded 30,899 deaths during September, the highest monthly figure of the year. The parishes within the walls suffered 15 per cent of plague deaths in the metropolis during the month, compared with fewer than 6 per cent during July, and far more were dying there of plague than in the Westminster parishes. But the worst affected areas were still those parishes around the walls, where between 40 and 50 per cent of all plague deaths were recorded during the summer months.

The high death toll had continued despite such practical measures as control of stray animals and fumigation of houses, and the medical help that was available. The corporation was able to put in place a team of ten or eleven physicians headed by Nathaniel Hodges and Thomas Witherley. They not only attended the sick and advised the authorities on treatment, but were curious to establish what they could about the nature of the disease. This led George Thomson and others to perform an autopsy on the body of a youth who had died of plague and later to publish the results. Medical staff were appointed at the pest-houses: a surgeon at that built by the parish of St Giles-in-the-Fields and a physician at the one erected by St Martin-in-the-Fields. Some physicians succumbed to the disease, although the numbers are uncertain. Others left, apparently to avoid the epidemic, although Hodges justified their action on the basis that it was due 'not so much for their own preservation as the service of those whom they attend'. A similar argument was offered by Jonathan Goddard, the Gresham Professor of Physic.[61]

Members of the parish clergy also departed. Early in August the physician Peter Barwick wrote to Sancroft, who had retired to Tunbridge Wells to take the waters, telling him that the 'mouths of a slanderous generation' were criticising 'those that are with drawn both of your profession and ours'. Some of the clergy did stay in London throughout the worst of the epidemic, including Simon Patrick at St Paul's, Covent Garden, Richard Peirson at St Bride's, Fleet Street, who signed every page of the burial register, and Robert Breton, vicar of St Nicholas's, Deptford, who was commended by Evelyn for remaining.[62] But the problem was serious enough for the Bishop of London, Humphrey Henchman, to try to stem the tide by warning those clergy who had left that they would be

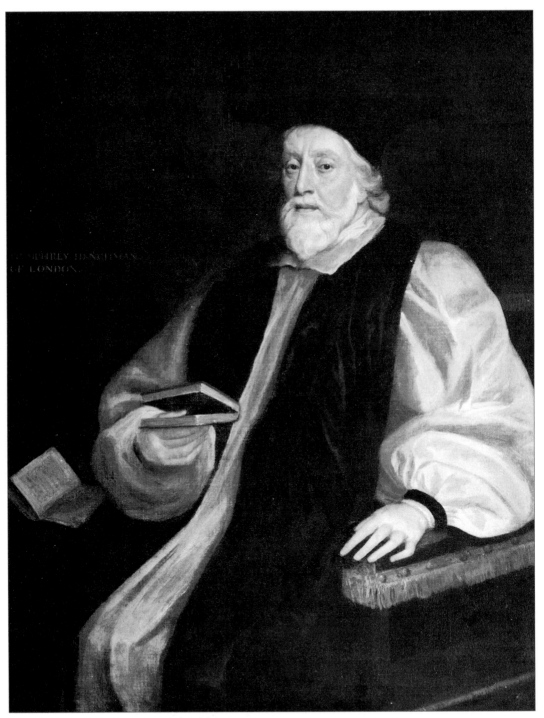

Humphrey Henchman, Bishop of London 1663–75, after Sir Peter Lely. (© Crown copyright, NMR)

replaced if they did not return. His anxiety was caused partly by a concern that nonconformist ministers would step in to conduct services where the Anglican clergy failed to meet the population's spiritual needs and maintain routines. These included conducting funerals and so observing the proper forms at a time when there were so many deaths. Not all of the parish clergy heeded Henchman's threats, and those who had moved away were censured in a pamphlet with the expressive title of *A Pulpit To Let*, which achieved considerable circulation.[63] Indeed, Henchman's fears were realised to a certain extent, for ministers who had lost their livings after the Restoration came back to the London pulpits, attracting large congregations. According to Gilbert Burnet, who was to become Bishop of Salisbury, they fulminated against the licentiousness of the court, as well as drawing attention to the way in which they had been treated by the Restoration regime. While their sermons were welcome to many citizens who remained in London, the size of the congregations was surely unfortunate at a time when crowds were likely to increase the spread of the disease. The clergy themselves were scarcely less at risk than the physicians and apothecaries in carrying out their duties: conducting services, officiating at funerals, receiving visitors from houses where the plague was present and having to go to the poor who were ill, to distribute alms. Of the Anglican clergy, at least eleven died of the plague, and some nonconformist preachers also expired, with six ministers recorded in the burial register of St Giles, Cripplegate.[64]

As the spiritual duties of the parishes came under strain, so did their administrative functions, with poor relief a growing and unavoidable expense. Some officers tried to move suspected plague victims out of their parish, to lessen the cost as well as to contain the outbreak, but the numbers involved must have made this impractical in many cases. The purchase by one parish of a sedan chair with restraining straps suggests that attempts were made to move the reluctant ones elsewhere, perhaps to a pest-house.[65] In social terms, the epidemic in 1665 followed the pattern of earlier plagues, with the poor particularly badly hit, while the wealthier citizens moved away, and so were not available to pay the rates levied to help the victims. Put succinctly, 'the rich hast away that should supply the pores want'.[66] Edmund Berry Godfrey, one of the Justices of the Peace for Westminster, complained that those who had gone away paid nothing. He regretted that the collectors of the plague and poor rates did not have the powers granted by Parliament to those gathering national taxation, which permitted them to force an entry and distrain goods for unpaid taxes.[67] By December less than half the sums due on the poor and plague rates had been received in some parishes. In such circumstances even the levying of extra rates was unlikely to produce money on the scale required. This was especially so in the less wealthy outer areas, where the crisis was far greater than in the City.

The shortfall in revenue from the rates was partly made up by voluntary donations from individuals, such as Sancroft, who sent money that was divided among the officers of a number of parishes for them to distribute to those in need. Simon Patrick was given £50 by just one benefactor for the sufferers in his parish and £10 by the Earl of Bedford, who donated a further £10 to help the victims in Westminster. Edward Wood instructed John Pack to give the needy poor in his parish up to 2s 6d each, but when he discovered that in four weeks only 4s 6d had been paid in all he told him to donate £5 to the churchwardens for them to distribute. The authorities at St Margaret's, Westminster received £1,652 for plague victims during the year, £1,117 of which was from such contributions by 'honourable persons'.[68] In addition, charitable collections across the country, with those taken on the fast days, supplied a relief fund from which £7,664 was distributed between July and December, and the Lord Mayor requested the livery companies to give towards poor relief one-third of the sums saved by the discontinuation of their feasts and other entertainments.[69] The City itself was generally able to meet the crisis. The aldermen authorised the levying of two extra years' poor rates and the chamberlain paid £600 per week during the summer to support parishes where the plague was present. The vestry of St Alphage's, London Wall collected £53 4s from its plague rate, but received £70 from the City. In these circumstances, it was agreed that money raised outside the City should be directed to the outer parishes.[70]

The problem of providing for the poor and the growing numbers of orphans was greatly increased by the policy of shutting up houses when plague was suspected, for those so confined had to be supplied with provisions. This became a major worry to the authorities, who were aware of the threat posed not only by the plague but also 'the want of Necessaries for life'.[71] Neighbours who could have provided help to those held in quarantine were likely to move away in alarm, afraid both of catching the disease and of finding their own houses closed. The more houses that were shut up and the greater the mortality, the fewer were the numbers able to help those confined to their houses. In an alley off Fleet Street, almost half the households were closed at some stage during the epidemic, and there were thirty-six deaths among the twenty houses.[72] Concern was aroused both in terms of the difficulties of providing aid on the large and increasing scale required, and because of the fear that it could lead to disorder, with those who

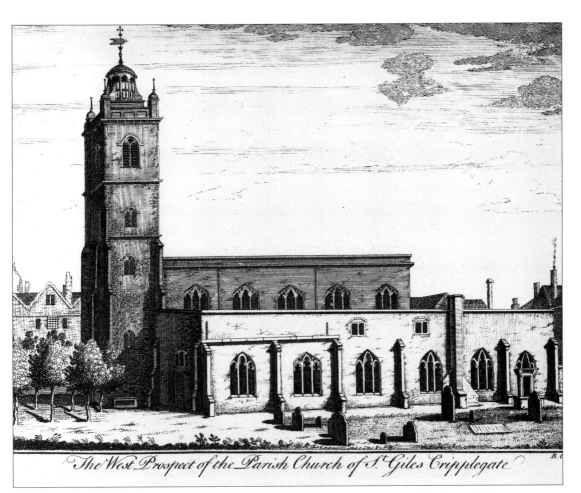

The West Prospect of the Parish Church of St Giles Cripplegate

The church of St Giles Cripplegate in the eighteenth century. The parish suffered very high mortality during the Great Plague. (© Crown copyright, NMR)

were immured being compelled to break out in order to search for food. In practice, the policy of sequestration seems to have been gradually abandoned for economic reasons and the shortage of people able and willing to undertake the duties of watching and nursing in the growing number of infected houses, rather than because of anxieties about disorder. By the middle of August the numbers infected in St Giles, Cripplegate were so great that the parish could not deal with the problem and so stopped confining plague suspects to their houses, 'least the sick & poore should be famished within dores'. A month later Pepys visited the Exchange, but spoke to as few people as possible, 'there being now no observation of shutting up houses of infected'. Thomas Vincent, too, noted that the shutting up of plague houses came to an end, 'there being so many'.[73]

Added to the fear of hunger and neglect felt by those who were quarantined was anxiety about the behaviour of the nurses who attended them. A harsh critic of the system of confinement described them as 'the off-scouring of the city' who were 'possessed with rooking avarice', watching for an opportunity to ransack the houses of their patients. Nathaniel Hodges was no less severe on the conduct of such nurses than on that of the apothecaries, asserting that they were 'barbarous wretches' who stole from those in their care. He also believed that they wilfully spread the disease, in order to increase the number of victims from whom they could steal, and even alleged that some had strangled their patients. The searchers who examined the bodies to establish the cause of death were also accused of pilfering from the houses of the plague victims.[74] Such thieving was all the more reprehensible in contemporaries' eyes because the circulation of goods stolen from those with plague was thought to be a means by which the disease was spread.

Attendance at funerals was also considered irresponsible, showing disregard for the common good. In mid-July the Lord Mayor, Sir John Lawrence, directed the aldermen to take greater care to prevent public funerals within the City, but they were not successful. A few weeks later, Clarendon, irritated by the failure to stop the practice and believing that the magistrates should use 'all force & rigour', wrote to Lawrence to demand greater efforts.[75] As the numbers of deaths continued to rise, at the end of August L'Estrange pointed to 'the incorrigible license of the multitudes that resort to publick funerals' as one of the causes. Pepys, too, commented on the numbers going to burials, with forty or fifty mourners at funerals that he saw in Southwark early in September. While such behaviour may have reflected a desire to continue to observe the normal rituals, he attributed it to sheer perversity, a defiance of the ban on funeral processions and assemblies, and agreed with members of the parish vestry at Greenwich to take some measures to prevent it. The lutenist and composer William Smegergill, who remained in Westminster throughout the year, thought that attendance at funerals was done 'in sport' by those taking risks out of sheer bravado.[76]

Pepys was also aware of the beggars in the streets. In October in Kent Street, 'a miserable, wretched, poor place' leading out of Southwark, he saw people begging, 'sitting sick and muffled up with plasters'.[77] A rise in the number of beggars was a consequence of the increasing inability to provide for the poor and effectively assist the plague victims. Evelyn went through the city on business during October and whenever he got out of his coach he found himself 'invironed with multitudes of poore pestiferous creatures, begging almes'.[78] In the previous month, while William Taswell's parents and his elder brother were lying ill at their house in Greenwich, he was ordered by his father to take some letters to London. Protected by angelica and 'some aromatics', the reluctant Taswell duly made his way to the city, where he encountered 'distressed objects . . . some under the direct influence of the plague, others lame through swellings, others again beckoning to me, and some carrying away upon biers to be buried'.[79]

Burials of victims should have been inconspicuous, as the plague orders directed that they should be conducted only during the hours of darkness. This system gradually broke down as the numbers increased, with too many dying each day for all the corpses to be interred during the short summer nights.

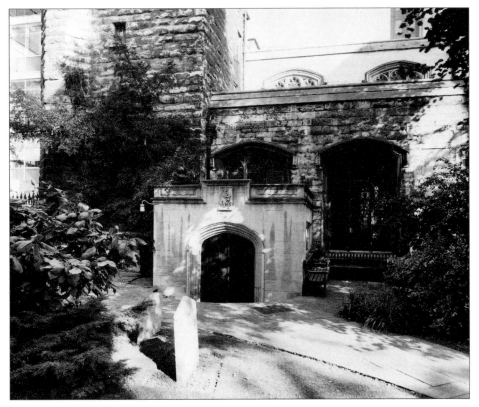

Samuel Pepys noted that the surface of the churchyard at St Olave, Hart Street, had risen during the epidemic, because of the number of burials there. It is now at a higher level than the church. (© Crown copyright, NMR)

At St Bride's there were more than thirty burials per day at the height of the epidemic. Furthermore, parish officers were faced with the problem of finding space in their churchyards and burial grounds, many of which were crowded already. In St Dunstan-in-the-West individual interments were replaced by burials in common graves from mid-August, and St Bride's adopted the same practice shortly afterwards. These two parishes had to dispose of 958 and 2,111 corpses respectively during the year, but the problem was even greater at St Botolph, Aldgate where 4,926 deaths were recorded, almost seven times the average annual number. There the parish had resort to a 'great pit', into which 1,114 bodies were placed. As the parishes began to fill their burial grounds they arranged for interments in the available space in the New Churchyard at Bethlem. Pepys was shocked to see how the graves lay 'so high upon the churchyard' of St Olave, Hart Street, at the end of the epidemic, yet more than 48 of the 194 burials from the parish during the year were in the New Churchyard, which was where at least 150 of the 355 whose deaths were recorded at St Benet, Paul's Wharf, were buried. But even the capacity of the New Churchyard was not enough, for the City acquired another 'new burial place' at Bunhill Fields, that was walled around by the middle of October.[80] A burial ground was also provided at the pest-house in Soho Fields. At the height of the plague the bodies were placed in pits, with up to forty in a pit, but as the number of deaths decreased individual graves were dug.[81]

The use of mass graves was dictated not only by the difficulties of finding space, but also by the need to bury the corpses as quickly as possible, to reduce the risk of the infection spreading. This was made more urgent by a shortage of coffins. The officers at St Bride's seem to have stopped placing bodies in them from the last week of July, suggesting that only shrouds were used. Many families could not pay the burial fees, which were received for only 17 per cent of interments during August, September and October. The organisation necessary for rapid burials was made more difficult by the high mortality among the parish officers. Both of the churchwardens at St Bride's and three churchwardens and the clerk of St Giles, Cripplegate died during the epidemic.[82] Yet in the intramural parish of St Thomas-the-Apostle rapid disposal of the dead was achieved. There were 152 burials in the second half of 1665, eleven times the average for the previous twenty years. Although this must have placed considerable pressure on the parish administration, all of the burials recorded after the end of June took place either on the day of death or during the following one. In non-plague years more than a third of interments there were on the

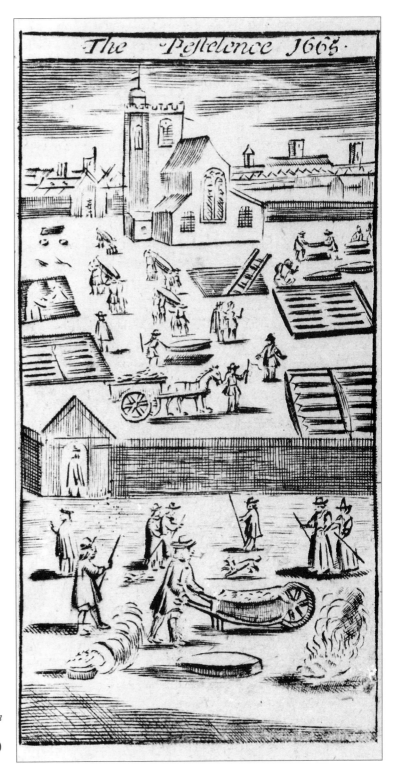

This drawing shows the orderly arrangement of burial spaces within mass graves. (© Guildhall Library, Corporation of London)

second day after death or following a longer interval.[83] Nevertheless, across the city, so many coffins had to be dealt with that some were left in the streets, awaiting collection.[84]

Londoners were also made aware of the high mortality from hearing the frequent passing of the carts collecting the corpses and the mournful tolling of the church bells. The carts were all the more intrusive because of the behaviour of their crews, which offended Thomas Rugg. He noted that many of them were 'very idle base liveing men and very rude' who drew attention to their task by 'swearing and cursing'. To John Allin the 'dolefull and almost universall and continuall ringing and tolling of bells' was an indication of the scale of the epidemic.[85]

Even for those who, like Oldenburg, had sealed themselves away and so avoided much unpleasantness, there was no escaping the sound of the bells. Yet he seems to have succeeded in being somewhat detached from the disaster. By the third week in August the only person known to him who had died was an under-postmaster, who 'lived closely and nastily' and, perhaps more significantly, had 'all sorts of people' calling on him to bring him letters.[86] Others, less secluded, knew of far more cases. Thomas Vincent later thought that he had heard of the death of someone known to him on almost every day for at least a month, and that perhaps as many as three-quarters of those he was used to seeing regularly had died during the epidemic. At the end of September Simon Patrick could think of ten clergymen who had died. A tenant of Dean Sancroft's, reported to be well on 18 August, died five days later and within three more weeks his entire family was said to have been 'swept away', except for one maid. Pepys heard that his baker 'with his whole family' had died, as had Will Griffith, an alehouse-keeper, his wife and three children, 'all I think in a day'.[87] Taswell visited a house where the mother was the sole survivor in the family, all seven of her children dying of the plague.[88] These may have been unusual cases, however, for a sample of six parishes shows that in almost two-thirds of affected households there was only one death, and that in only one-twentieth were there more than three deaths. The pattern suggests that many households were infected, but typically lost only one or two members. The example of St Dunstan-in-the-West shows that at a more local level there was a contrast between the main streets, where single deaths were typical, and the alleys and courts, such as Cock and Key Alley, where there was an average of three deaths in each of the twelve infected houses.[89] This may reflect the fact that the wealthier citizens living in the principal thoroughfares were those who had gone away, leaving much-reduced households consisting of just one or two servants, to take care of the property. That is what Taswell's family did, entrusting the house to a 'good old faithful servant'. She contracted the plague, but recovered, and the only death in the house was that of a manservant.[90]

As the high mortality continued, conversations naturally included exchanges of information about who had died or been taken ill. Pepys found this a depressing aspect of going around London, noting at the end of August that 'everybody's looks and discourse in the street is of death and nothing else', and again later that he overheard 'so many sad stories . . . everybody talking of this dead, and that man sick, and so many in this place, and so many in that'. Lady Giffard, too, was dismayed by the almost constant reports of victims, with 'people coming in like Job's messengers all day, with one sad story before another was ended'.[91] Given the disruption of social intercourse, there was much uncertainty, leading to false

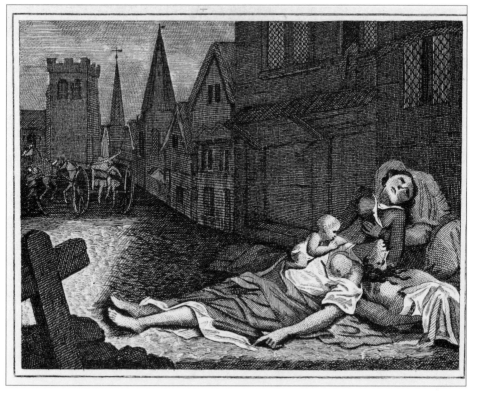

Robert Pollard's portrayal of London during the Great Plague shows two women lying dead in a street. (© Wellcome Institute Library, London)

reports. Patrick had to correct his list of deceased clergymen, for one minister reported dead was still alive, although his curate was not. He also discovered that the rector of St Andrew's, Holborn had not died but gone away.[92]

At times of uncertainty, sudden death and high anxiety, suspicions were quickly aroused. The house of Alexander Burnet, a physician, in Fenchurch Street was one of the first in the City to be infected with plague, his servant William Passon dying from the disease. Although Burnet was respected by his neighbours for reacting swiftly and causing the house to be shut up, a rumour spread that he had killed Passon, and this became so widely reported that the doctor felt compelled to place a denial in *The Intelligencer*. He also showed Pepys the note from the master of the pest-house certifying that Passon had a bubo on his groin and two spots on his thigh, providing clear evidence, as Pepys agreed, that he had died of the plague.[93]

Such swellings of the lymph nodes, commonly in the groin but perhaps in the armpit or on the neck, made the cause of death evident and were accepted by the searchers as proof of a plague death. John Allin's close friend Peter Smith died within four days of being taken ill, first having a fever and then developing a swelling under his ear. The other physical manifestation of plague was the appearance of large spots or blotches on the skin, known as the 'tokens'. Because of these blotches plague was described as the spotted disease, hence John Dryden's reference in *Annus Mirabilis* to the time 'When spotted death ran arm'd through every street'. The fever and neurological and psychological disturbances that the victim suffered were further characteristics of the plague, often producing delirium accompanied by erratic and uncontrollable behaviour and loud shrieks. The fear that the disease engendered was succinctly expressed by Allin in his comment that 'it is a greate mercy now counted to dye of another disease'.[94]

Unusually high numbers of deaths from other diseases were indeed recorded in the *Bills* throughout the period of the epidemic. This may have been due partly to lack of nursing because of a fear of going near anyone who was ill, in case plague was the cause. The disruption resulting from the conditions is likely to have increased the number of deaths among those who were vulnerable through age or illness, but it is improbable that it produced a thirtyfold increase in deaths from 'surfeit'. Specific cases also cast doubt on the reliability of some attributions. For example, it seems unlikely that 'dropsy' caused the death of the parish clerk of St Giles, Cripplegate – one of the worst affected parishes – and his wife, who died on the same day.[95] Deliberate misidentification of the cause of death, in order to reduce the number entered as attributable to plague, must partly account for the increase in non-plague deaths. The pattern of such deaths was similar to those from plague, with the weekly numbers steadily increasing until the end of August and beginning of September, when they were three times the level recorded in June and more than four times the average for that time of year. Fever and spotted fever accounted for 36 per cent of the 13,741 non-plague deaths entered in July, August and September, and consumption for a further 12 per cent. Those attributed to spotted fever during the summer months were twenty times higher than the average of recent years. The numbers for all three categories declined thereafter, as plague deaths fell, but those succumbing to fevers fell to 21 per cent of non-plague deaths, while the proportion of consumption victims remained at the same level.[96]

From 4,327 deaths from plague in the week ending 10 October there was a steady decrease, to just 1,031 four weeks later. However, the growing optimism was checked by the returns for the next week, 1–7 November, when there was a sharp rise to 1,414 plague deaths, news which, as Pepys noted, 'makes us all sad'. He had expected an increase during the previous week, which in fact had seen a fall of 390 plague deaths, although without noting a reason for his pessimism. The increase was attributed to a premature return by some of those who had left

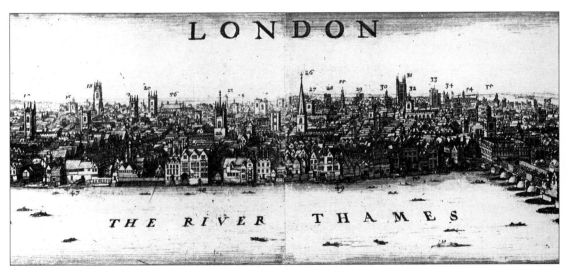

Wenceslaus Hollar's view of the City in the mid-seventeenth century shows it as densely built up. Nevertheless, mortality during the Great Plague was lower there than in other parts of the metropolis. (© Crown copyright, NMR)

earlier, increasing the size of the population at risk from infection. Those who returned to London doubtless wished to get back to normal as soon as possible, with economic necessity overriding their caution, and they may also have been concerned by the vulnerability of their empty premises to burglary. Rugg made a note that 'many thieves rob houses' and described a case where burglars had broken into a stocking cellar to steal silk stockings and fine linen, putting their booty into two coffins, hoping to get away unnoticed. Despite their resourcefulness, those would-be robbers were caught, but such stories were likely to alarm those who were away from home.[97]

The rise in plague deaths was also blamed on the unseasonably mild weather, but it proved to be short-lived, for the following week produced figures similar to those at the end of October, while the next return, ending 21 November, showed a sharp fall, from 1,050 deaths from plague to 652. Even so, the disease remained widespread, with 82 of the 130 parishes recording plague deaths during that week. It had been anticipated that cold winter weather would reduce the incidence of the disease and Pepys hoped that the frosty spell towards the end of November would bring 'a perfect cure of the plague'.[98] But this did not happen, for although the numbers of deaths from the disease continued to fall at the end of November and into December, they rose again in the second and third weeks of December. The four weeks following 22 November produced a combined total of 987 victims. During this period deaths from other diseases were below the normal level, but the plague deaths kept the total numbers of dead at more than 50 per cent above the decennial average.[99]

The decline in the numbers of plague victims was not greeted with universal relief, for clergymen who regarded the epidemic as a divine punishment felt that the burden was being lifted before the full lesson of the need to repent had been learned. That the plague was a judgement on a sinful people was an argument expounded by the clergy both in their weekly sermons and in those delivered on the monthly fast days. The logic of this point of view was that God controlled the extent of the disease. Thus, according to Simon Patrick, the increase at the beginning of November was due to His wise goodness, and should be interpreted as a warning, showing that 'wee are not yet so safe' as complacent sinners might imagine. Already there had been a falling off in the numbers in his congregation, and so the effect of the increase in the number of plague deaths after several weeks of decline might be to 'rouse up dull Souls'.[100]

The view of the Anglican hierarchy was indeed that plague should be seen as a punishment for sin that demonstrated the need for repentance. This was expressed in the *Form of Common Prayer* issued for use on the fast days, which also reflected the fear of widespread disorder, perhaps even rebellion. Among other texts, it drew attention to the passage in the book of Numbers which describes how a rebellion among the Israelites against Moses and Aaron was punished by God with a visitation of the plague. The connection between resistance to authority and the pestilence was clear. To emphasise the point, a parallel was drawn between the defiance of Moses and Aaron and those in England 'that strive both with their Princes and their Priests'. Traitors had dared to lift up their hands against the Lord's anointed, and so 'what wonder that there is wrath gone out from the Lord, and the Plague is begun?'. This could be interpreted as a reference to the events of the 1640s and 1650s, as well as a warning not to countenance rebellion against the Restoration regime, reflecting the government's apprehension of political disorder at a time of suspected plots and conspiracies.[101]

The threat posed by religious dissent could be lessened by the enforcement of the Conventicle Act, which provided for the imprisonment and transportation of those who attended nonconformists' religious meetings. Of the Quakers who were rounded up, fifty-two died of the plague in Newgate gaol and twenty-seven more while they were being held on a ship awaiting transportation. They were on board for seven months, by which time the vessel had got no further than Plymouth, where permission to land was refused, and she was captured by the Dutch as she finally set sail for the West Indies. To hold in check the more sinister elements in the capital, Albemarle had at his disposal a detachment of soldiers quartered in Hyde Park and the garrison of the Tower. Neither force escaped the plague, however, with fifty-eight of the soldiers from the Tower removed to a pest-house and a third of those in Hyde Park falling victim to the disease. Many of their officers fled to avoid the infection.[102]

Evelyn noted twenty-six sermons that he heard between 23 July and the end of the year. Both the texts and the explications reflected the senior Anglican clergy's interpretations of the epidemic. In his sermon on the fast day in October, Thomas Plume, vicar of Greenwich, drew on the *Form of Common Prayer* and preached on the plague sent among the Israelites for disobeying Moses and Aaron. Evelyn described the subject as 'the sinn of rebellion against Magistrates & Ministers'. Another of Plume's sermons addressed personal rather than political sinfulness, using a text from Colossians, which explicitly mentioned 'fornication, uncleanness, inordinate affection, evil concupiscence, and covetousness, which is idolatry' as bringing the wrath of God on the children of disobedience.

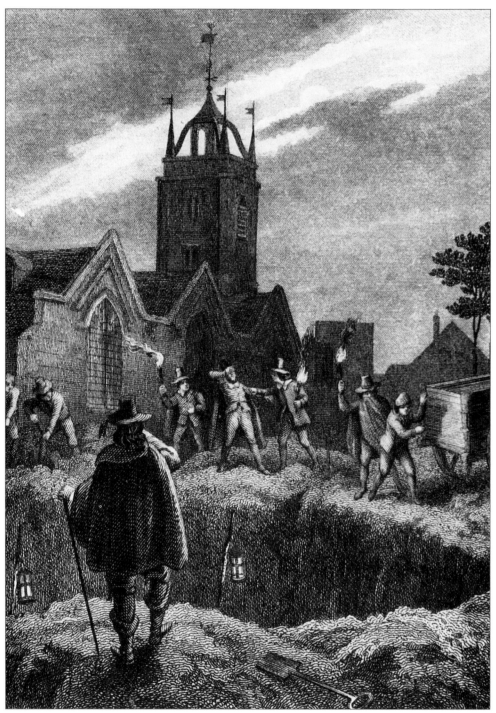

Bodies being buried in a pit at Aldgate, by George Cruikshank. (© Wellcome Institute Library, London)

It was not entirely a wrathful God who was portrayed from the pulpit, however, especially as the numbers of victims declined. John Higham, rector of Wotton, liked the analogy of the story of the Prodigal Son, which showed that those who repented would be forgiven, using it on 8 October and 19 November. The need for repentance had to be recognised from the warning of the plague, as did God's mercy and forgiveness, in limiting his anger by reducing the number of victims. But some of the population may not have realised that they should be penitent, being reassured by their own survival. The clergy were aware of the danger of smugness and false pride among those who survived, based on the assumption that the sinners had been taken. Evelyn particularly commended as 'a seasonable discourse' a sermon at Greenwich in December, when the preacher drew on a text from St Luke's gospel, which showed that those who died a sudden death were not 'sinners above all men', to make the point that those who had survived the plague should not condemn those who had not. Evelyn's own reaction to having lived through the year was to echo the words of Psalm 91, noting his thankfulness for His mercy 'when thousands & ten thousands perish'd and were swept away on each side of me'. He believed that he had been spared so that he would be able to 'recount & magnifie' God's goodness in allowing him to live.[103]

Edward Wood also praised God for 'his mercyfull preservation of us in the midst of soe greate contagion'. But he was aware that God's mercy should not be taken for granted, writing to John Pack that 'as tis not goode to distract gods power in protecting you soe tis not goode to tempt god too far'. Wood regarded the outbreak as God's punishment and a means to attempt to 'teach us righteousnes', using the image of a destroying angel controlled by the Almighty and praying that God would 'stay his hand & send health amongst us'. There is no reason to doubt Wood's sincerity or his faith, yet his letters to Pack moved seamlessly from such sentiments to the practicalities of their trade in commodities.[104] Pepys's survey of the plague months was even more secular, for he noted that the epidemic had cost him money, in having to maintain separate households at Woolwich and London and his clerks at Greenwich. This was alleviated on 6 January, when his wife returned to Seething Lane. By then there was a general movement back to the metropolis, Pepys noticing that by the end of December 'the town fills apace'. Even Daniel Milles, the rector of St Olave, Hart Street had returned by the first Sunday in February, being castigated by Pepys for leaving the parish before anyone else 'and now staying till all are come home'. Pepys's irritation was more than matched by those who had provided hospitality

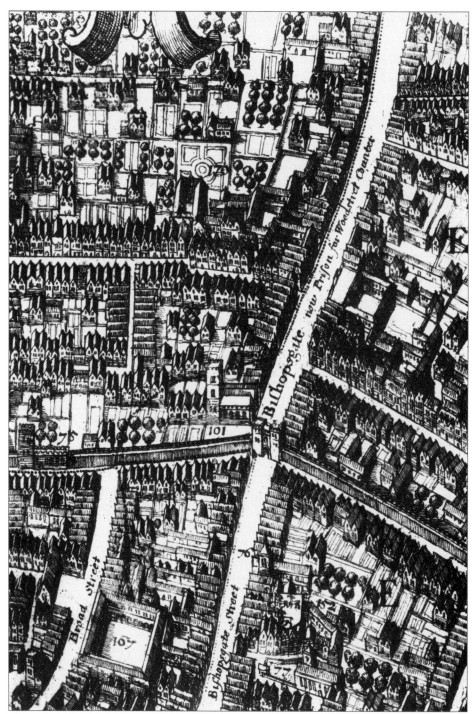

Wenceslaus Hollar's plan-view of the Bishopsgate area at the time of the plague. (© Crown copyright, NMR)

for apprentices who had been left behind, but who were unable to recover the costs from their masters when they had returned. Simon Romney's apprentice William Law had lived with Francis Taylor, a cook, during Romney's absence in the country, and had died in Taylor's house. Yet Romney refused to pay not only the costs of Law's board and lodging, but also those of his funeral, and had to be sued by Taylor for payment.[105]

There was a scare in December when the *Bills* showed a steady increase in deaths from plague. However, when the weather turned cold enough for ice to form on the Thames, it was assumed that the numbers would fall again. But Pepys was concerned that if that did not happen the disease would continue into 1666. Evelyn, too, was cautious and even in the middle of January he was unwilling to bring his wife and family back to Deptford. They eventually moved there early in February, and Richard Baxter returned to Acton a month later. The most significant return of all was that of the king to Whitehall on 1 February, bringing a restoration of something close to normality for those who were economically dependent on the court.[106]

Pepys's apprehensions for the coming year were realised, for although the numbers of plague victims declined, a few dozen burials were returned each week. During March and April the weekly average was only thirty plague burials, but the first three weeks of May brought a steady rise. Yet this increase did not cause the alarm that a similar rise had produced in the previous year, and the numbers decreased again. Throughout June, July and August the average weekly return was thirty-six, with a high point of fifty-one in mid-July, and the number of parishes with plague deaths peaked at twenty-one in the second week in August. Almost 1,800 plague burials were recorded during 1666, making it the worst year for the disease in London since 1647, with the spectacular exception of 1665.[107]

The annual *Bill* for 1665 covered the period 27 December 1664 to 19 December 1665, during which there had been 97,306 deaths, 68,596 of them attributed to plague. Contemporaries were sceptical of the numbers of plague deaths recorded, Clarendon speculating that the true figure had been 160,000. His estimate is implausibly high, yet is indicative of the lack of confidence in the figures presented in the *Bill*. The average number of burials over the previous ten years had been 16,600 per year. Graunt and Petty made estimates of the death rate in London that ranged between 31.2 and 34.1 per 1,000, excluding plague victims. In 1665, by contrast, the death rate was 195 per 1,000, in a population estimated at 500,000.[108] The figures are not entirely comparable, because the

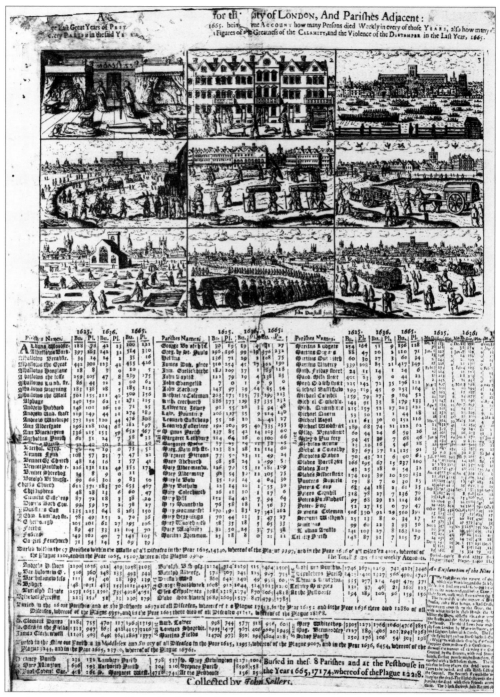

A contemporary broadsheet showing the figures for the numbers of deaths recorded in the Bills of Mortality *during 1665, and scenes associated with the epidemic, including the killing of animals, the departure and return of the citizens, and burials.* (© Museum of London)

population of London was somewhat smaller during the second half of 1665, partly because of those who had left to avoid the epidemic, and partly due to the number of deaths. In addition, the problems of maintaining an accurate record were much greater during the plague, because of disrupted parochial administration and the sheer scale of the operation in some parishes during the worst weeks.

The actual number of plague deaths is difficult to estimate. The 'expected' number of burials of 16,600 has to be adjusted to take account of the shrunken population from July to December. A rate assessment for Westminster in September suggests that 12 per cent of the inhabitants had left. Applying this proportion to the whole city for the second half of the year, but with a 'normal' mortality rate for the first six months, reduces the 'expected' number of burials for the year to 15,600. Subtracting this from the total in the *Bill* produces a figure of 81,700 for the 'excess' deaths, the majority of which were caused by plague and were either entered as such or were concealed under other categories. But it cannot be assumed that all of the 'excess' deaths attributed to such categories were in fact concealed plague deaths, for the patterns of burials within the parishes suggest upsurges of other diseases during the summer, although the proportion of 'false' and 'true' attributions cannot be recovered.

Further deaths went unrecorded because some victims may have left London after contracting plague and died elsewhere, and not all of the population lay within the parochial system. The Jewish community was so reduced in numbers by departures and deaths that in the spring of 1666 attendance at the synagogue was 'much diminished'. The Quakers recorded 1,177 deaths during the year, and according to contemporaries, burials of members of other nonconformist sects took place 'whereof no churchwarden or other officer had notice'.[109] Parish registers record the reading of the burial service, not the names of all those who had died, and so some of those outside the Anglican Church may not have been enumerated in the *Bills*. This is suggested by a comparison of the numbers entered in the registers of eight City parishes with their returns in the Bills, which in seven cases shows little variation between the two sets of figures. In other words, the numbers in the *Bills* were a record of those buried according to the rites of the Anglican Church. The only exception in the sample is Allhallows, London Wall where 333 burials are listed in the register, but the *Bills* have the much higher, and suspiciously round, figure of 500. The discrepancy between the two figures suggests that the parochial system may have broken down during the epidemic and the number of deaths in the *Bills* is

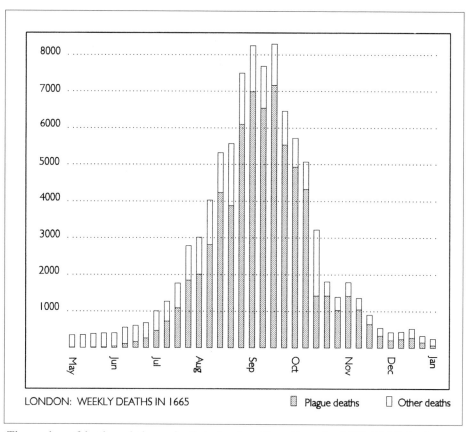

The numbers of deaths and plague-deaths in London, May–December 1665. (© Michael Clements)

an estimate.[110] Furthermore, deaths within the seven liberties outside the parish system were not included in the *Bills*.

Despite its imperfections, the evidence suggests an estimate of more than 70,000, and perhaps as many as 75,000, deaths from plague. This represented roughly 15 per cent of the population, and 17 per cent of those citizens remaining in London in the second half of 1665. Allowing for those deaths which went unrecorded in the Bills, it is possible that the total number exceeded 100,000, or perhaps 20 per cent of the inhabitants and a sixfold increase on the decennial annual average.

The overall total conceals variations in the chronology and distribution of the epidemic. The peak in the number of burials in St Giles-in-the-Fields, which was the first parish to be infected on a large scale, came in late July 1665, but in

St Andrew, Holborn and St James, Clerkenwell, the high point was towards the end of August. In St Giles, Cripplegate the worst week came in mid-August, and by the third week in September the numbers had fallen to only a little over half those buried at the peak, while in St Botolph, Bishopsgate the greatest number of deaths was in the week ending 5 September, and in Stepney the first three weeks of September produced the highest mortality of the epidemic. But the pattern cannot be interpreted simply in terms of the disease moving steadily eastwards from a source in the west of the city, for burials in Westminster also peaked in September.[111]

The intensity of the epidemic also varied. The worst affected areas lay around the edge of the City: to the west, in St Andrew, Holborn and St Giles-in-the-Fields; to its north, in St Giles, Cripplegate, St Leonard, Shoreditch and St Botolph, Bishopsgate; to the east, in St Botolph, Aldgate, Whitechapel and Stepney; and, across the Thames, in Southwark.[112] By the 1660s the suburbs

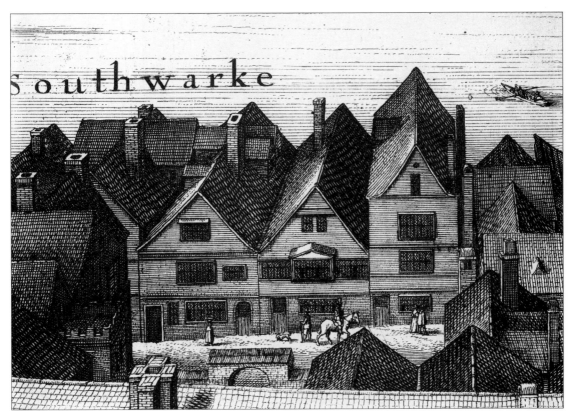

A closely built area of Southwark, which suffered high mortality during the plague, shown in Wenceslaus Hollar's view. (© Crown copyright, NMR)

south of the Thames, including Southwark, had a population of approximately 50,000 and 15,533 deaths were recorded there in 1665, or roughly 30 per cent of the inhabitants. Dividing the number of deaths by the annual average over the previous decade produces a multiple, or crisis mortality ratio, of 6.4 for this area. By contrast, the ninety-seven parishes within the city walls escaped relatively lightly, for although there were 15,207 deaths, the crisis mortality ratio was only 4.6. Indeed, those parishes which experienced the smallest increases in numbers of burials in 1665 were generally clustered around Cheapside, in the wealthiest part of the metropolis.

But not all of the badly stricken areas were outside the walls, for a group of four parishes just inside them, in the north-east of the City, had levels of mortality that were almost eight times the average, amongst the highest in the capital. Adjoining them, but beyond the walls, there were 8,390 deaths in St Botolph, Aldgate and St Botolph, Bishopsgate, compared with the annual average of 1,231, a crisis mortality ratio of 6.8, slightly higher than the 6.5 in the outer East End parishes of Whitechapel and Stepney, which had 13,364 deaths. Whitechapel and Stepney were large and relatively poor, with an average of 2.7 hearths per household, as assessed for the hearth tax, and a high proportion of householders who were exempt from paying the tax because of their poverty, with as many as 70 per cent in Whitechapel falling into that category. The comparable figure in St Andrew, Holborn and St Giles-in-the-Fields, to the west of the City, was approximately 25 per cent, and those parishes experienced 8,415 deaths, 5.7 times the annual average.[113]

Generally, there was an inverse relationship between wealth and mortality, with the richest parishes suffering the least impact during the year. The twelve parishes with the lowest crisis mortality ratios had 5.9 hearths per household, while the average household in the twelve parishes with the highest such ratios had 2.8 hearths. The parishes in these samples were also markedly different in their population size, however, for the wealthier ones were small, while the twelve worst-affected ones were on average fifteen times more populous, and so contained a much greater range of household types. A similar contrast in wealth and death rates is apparent between the extensive parishes of St Giles, Cripplegate and St Leonard, Shoreditch, north of the City, where the mean number of hearths per household was 2.9, and Westminster, where the comparable figure was 5.0 hearths. The 10,738 deaths in St Giles and St Leonard produced a crisis mortality ratio of 7.2, compared with 4.7 in Westminster, where 12,194 deaths were recorded. The effects of the plague broadly reflected the distribution of wealth within the metropolis.[114]

According to Clarendon's assessment of the Great Plague in London, 'The greatest number of those who died consisted of women and children, and the lowest and poorest sort of the people', to which he added that 'not many of wealth or quality or of much conversation' had been killed. John Gadbury wrote in similar terms, that the plague destroyed the 'dregs' of society, but that the more 'noble' part of the population survived.[115] Despite the crudity of these summaries, in social terms they seem to have been broadly correct. The ability to move away from London in time undoubtedly reduced the number of deaths among the well-to-do, and to that extent the *Bills* served their purpose, by providing a warning of the coming and escalation of the epidemic. In the wealthy areas, therefore, a high proportion of those who died during the epidemic were poor, their better-off neighbours having left. But even within a relatively poor parish such as St Giles, Cripplegate, in an area where the economy was dominated by small craftsmen, 30 per cent of the burials between June and December 1665 in which the occupational category was recorded were those of servants and labourers.[116] Nevertheless, the plague had claimed victims from many sections of society. They included Sir Thomas Noell, a prominent merchant and former MP, Peter Llewellyn, who had been under-clerk of the Council of State, John Bide, an alderman for four years in the 1650s, and two of the members of Westminster Abbey choir.[117] Among the artistic community there had been the death in 1665 of the sculptor John Colt the younger, in St Bartholomew the Great, which was probably attributable to plague, and Wenceslaus Hollar's only son was certainly a victim, and a sad loss, for he was described as 'an ingeniose youth, drew delicately'.[118]

Clarendon's reference to the deaths of women and children also needs to be modified, although it was not without some truth, so far as the impact on the female population was concerned. London contained more males than females, and so in normal years male deaths exceeded those of females. In contrast, the pattern for 1665 shows slightly more female than male deaths over the whole year, and during the months of epidemic the mortality rate among females increased more than it did among males. Before the outbreak there were 130 male burials for every 100 female ones in the parish of St Thomas the Apostle and 88 male burials for every 100 female burials in St Olave, Old Jewry. During the epidemic these ratios were markedly different, with just 104 male burials per 100 female burials in St Thomas's and 55 in St Olave's. The two parishes had a different population structure, with males in the majority in St Thomas's and females in St Olave's, yet in both the proportion of female deaths was much higher during the plague. This pattern occurred in both rich and poor parishes. It may be that, in the wealthier ones at least, the composition of the population changed somewhat during the epidemic, with women housekeepers remaining behind in houses left almost empty. The vulnerability of domestic servants may also account for the death rate among females, in having to go to public places to buy provisions, and to run other errands. The evidence for the impact on children is much less certain because of the inconsistencies in recording them, although it seems unlikely that there was an upsurge in deaths among the young during the plague.[119]

The Great Plague in London undoubtedly was a shocking experience that touched all of the city's inhabitants in differing degrees. Pepys saw a great deal of the consequences of the epidemic, yet could write at the end of the year that none of his immediate family or friends had died, perhaps forgetting that his aunt, Edith Bell of the parish of St Bartholomew-the-Less, and his physician had been among the victims. Thomas Rugg was even more detached, making entries in his journal regarding the progress of the disease and its effects, but no reference to the death of anyone known to him. Anselm Herford had come much closer to death, and looked back with relief and gratitude that he had survived, when the entire family he had been lodging with had not.[120] To the Earl of Clarendon, who spent the second half of the year away from London, it meant a frustrating separation from friends, prompting him to ask 'Are wee alwayes to be separated and never meete agayne?' The disruption of which he wrote was a consequence of dispersal; to many families it was brought by death. In St Giles, Cripplegate, Felix Bragg, his wife and daughter were buried on the same day; four children from one family were interred within six days; and in the space of four days the parish clerk recorded the burials of Thomas Crawley, his wife, son, two daughters and a journeyman who worked for him.[121] Experiences such as these made up a complex pattern of death and upheaval, concentrated into seven months, varying between households and from one part of the capital to another. Other diseases may have contributed, but plague was the predominant killer in an epidemic that produced more deaths in London in a single year than ever before.

CHAPTER 3
The Plague in the Provinces

The wrath of the Lord was kindled against the people, and the Lord smote
the people with a very great plague.

Numbers, 11:33

We acknowledge indeed, that our punishments are less than our deservings;
but yet of thy mercy, O Lord, correct us to amendment and plague us not to
our destruction.

A Form of Common Prayer, together With an Order of Fasting, for the Averting
of God's heavy Visitation (1665)

An outbreak of plague in London was bound to cause alarm throughout the
country, for experience in past epidemics had shown that it was likely to spread
elsewhere. The capital's importance in the national economy and cultural life was
such that it lay at the hub of the networks of internal trade and social travel, and it
was by far the most important port. Movement between provincial communities
and London brought the risk of infection, yet was difficult to control and
potentially harmful to stop, for to cease contact with the metropolis would be to
risk causing economic dislocation. Nor was London the only source of danger, for
communities could be infected independently, with the ports on the east and south
coasts particularly at risk from plague that was being spread along the trade routes
of northern Europe. In addition to the normal intercourse, an epidemic produced
migration away from an infected community that involved movement of people on
an unusually large scale within a short space of time, perhaps including some who
already had the disease. While the plague was confined to London and a few other
towns, regulation of travellers who might pose a risk was possible, but when it
spread more widely, such controls became increasingly difficult to maintain.

Despite the problems and possible effects, with the news of the outbreak in
London in the early summer of 1665 the authorities in many towns put measures
in place to attempt to keep their communities free from plague. These were

based upon regulations that had been applied before. The justices at Hereford were concerned with the cleanliness of the streets, ordering the removal of piles of rubbish and instructing householders with pumps to use them to flush down the gutters and channels for half an hour daily during hot weather. Pigs were to be kept 'up close in the house' or taken out of the city. The justices particularly feared the risk posed by the carriers who travelled to and from London, and the passengers who they brought back with them.[1] Those at Leicester shared that concern and ordered that carriers should no longer go to London; if any continued to do so then they must find lodgings and places to air their goods, some distance from the town. The orders issued in 1625 regarding the reception of anyone coming from London were consulted and a ruling made that nobody from the capital, or any other infected place, was to be allowed into the town unless they had the permission of the mayor or the justices. Their decision was to be made on the credit they gave to the certificate of health held by the traveller. Huts were built outside the town to provide accommodation for those who were excluded by these measures.[2] At York, innkeepers were instructed to report new arrivals in the city to the mayor.[3] The justices at Lincoln assizes directed the petty constables to apprehend vagrants and 'wandering persons', to examine other travellers and strangers, and to prevent them from taking accommodation unless they could demonstrate that they were free from infection, presumably by producing a health certificate. In October a system of

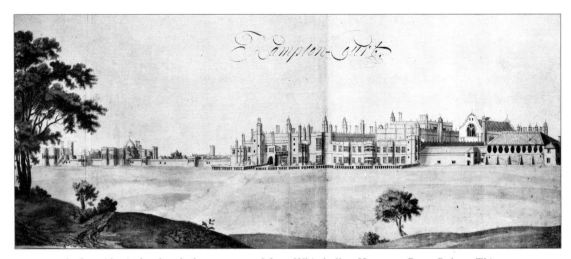

As the epidemic developed, the court moved from Whitehall to Hampton Court Palace. This view dates from 1669. (© Crown copyright, Historic Royal Palaces)

guards to patrol the streets was instituted in the city.[4] Preventive action of this kind appears to have been taken by many local authorities in the wake of the news from London, with the issue of orders aimed at the cleanliness of public places, the exclusion of those who were regarded as a risk, and the introduction of health certificates for travellers.

Some of those who left London to escape the plague went a considerable distance. Griffith Bodurda went to Wales, for instance, and the Radcliffe family to Northumberland, while Mary Walker, a servant, obtained a health certificate from the churchwardens of St Andrew Undershaft and moved to Evesham.[5] Her hand-written certificate was accepted, but confidence in such documents was undermined by the appearance of forgeries. The problem was such that the officers of London parishes placed advertisements in the newspapers in an attempt to restore the credibility of the system. One issued by the churchwardens of St Gregory's in July 1665 stated that they gave certificates only to those known to them to be free from plague, and that all such documents emanating from them were printed. Warnings of potential carriers of the disease were also published. Consequently, those who had left London after having been in contact with a plague victim, and so lacking a certificate, could not be sure that they would remain unidentified. When the maid of an upholsterer in Covent Garden died, he and several others living in the house left, taking some possessions with them, but a notice in *The London Gazette* gave their names and ordered that a search should be made for them, so that the justices could close the houses where they lodged.[6]

The fear of those arriving from London or another place where the plague was known to have erupted was intensified by outbreaks that could be attributed to suspect persons from outside the community. Following the death of a man from plague in Walsall in August 1665, regulations controlling access were put in place, partly because it was realised that carriers were being tempted by the sums they were paid for bringing passengers and goods to the town from infected areas. The appearance of plague in Lichfield in the following month was blamed on the 'covetousness' of a family who had lodged travellers from the capital who were carrying the disease. In turn, the authorities at Coventry were alarmed by the risk that plague could be brought from Lichfield and a report in October described how 'a disorderly fellow entertained an infected person in an ale-house in the suburbs: whereupon the master of the house died'.[7] This account encapsulates the characteristic anxiety of the authorities that some people were careless, or even predisposed to ignore regulations, and so could put the whole community at risk, and these were commonly regarded as being the frequenters of alehouses and the inhabitants of the suburbs. Fear bred harshness, even cruelty, to those who were suspected as carriers of plague. Henry Newcome even refused to take in his own cousin, who had come from London to Lancashire to stay with him, justifying his action on the grounds that it had been ordered that neither people or goods should be received without the constable's permission. Newcome asked his cousin to stay in an inn until he could speak with the constable, but, after this rebuff, he took umbrage 'and after would not come to me'. In November 1665 John Overing wrote from London to William Sancroft at Tunbridge Wells, excusing himself from going there in person partly because of 'the unkindnesse of country people to Londoners'. Such treatment produced a reaction in London, expressed in an indignant report carried by *The Intelligencer* in September, that a man who arrived at Dorchester from London was accommodated in a shed in a field, where he died within four days, and then a pit was dug so that 'both hovel and corpse were buried together'.[8]

Those communities around the city were most immediately at risk from refugees carrying the disease. In October 1665 James Hickes, the postmaster, wrote that he did not know of anywhere near London that was not infected.[9]

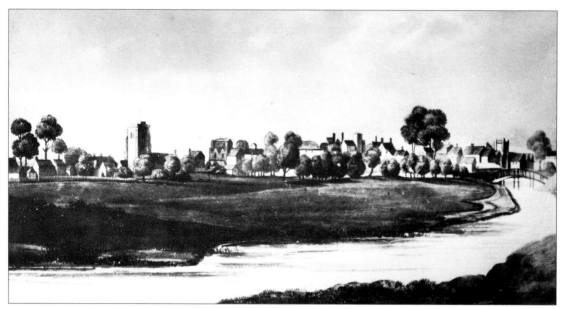

Brentford suffered heavily during the plague epidemic. This view dates from c. 1660. (© Crown copyright, NMR)

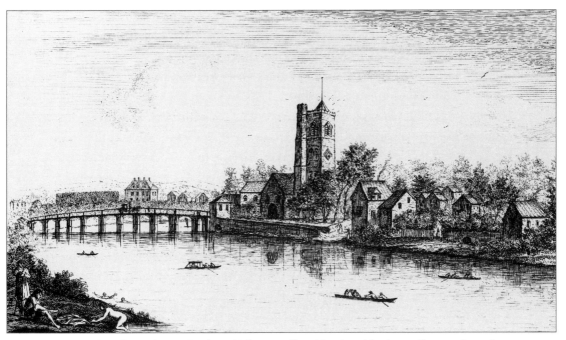

Among the villages close to London which were affected by the epidemic was Putney, shown here in a view of 1738. (© B.T. Batsford Ltd)

Hampstead's position on high ground had gained it the reputation of having clear, healthy air, and so it was bound to attract people from London trying to avoid the plague yet not willing to go far away. The consequence was 260 deaths in 100 houses during 1665, although the population was only approximately 800 in normal conditions.[10]

The epidemic also made a considerable impact in the communities along the Thames upstream from London. There were 122 deaths from the disease at Kingston-upon-Thames during 1665, and at Brentford more than 300 plague deaths were reported by the first week in October, with 432 noted in the burial register by the end of the year. Steps taken at Brentford to alleviate the suffering met with opposition, producing the complaint that 'the richer will not contribute, nor the meaner submit, though for their own preservation'. The churchwardens at Putney employed a dog-catcher to deal with strays, but their efforts were in vain, and seventy-four plague burials were recorded in the parish during the year. Wandsworth's register included 245 plague deaths, in a parish with roughly 340 houses. The first burial of a plague victim at Croydon may have taken place in mid-June, although not until 27 July was a death attributed to the disease recorded in the parish register. Interments rose during September and peaked in October, with the last recorded plague burial taking place on 17 March 1666. The isolation offered by an almshouse did not provide security here, for six of the inmates of the Whitgift hospital died in the epidemic, among a total of 141 deaths from plague. Yet other places, nearer to the city, escaped relatively lightly. Only twenty-eight plague deaths were recorded at Kensington in 1665 and fifteen in the following year, and the total number of deaths was just 50 per cent higher than the decennial average.[11]

The inhabitants of the towns and villages close to London who felt themselves to be in danger reacted accordingly. When Pepys visited Lady Wright's house near Dagenham in Essex in mid-July he found that 'all these great people here are afeared of London, being doubtful of anything that comes from thence or that hath lately been there'. Their concern was such that he felt it prudent to lie about his arrangements, assuring them that he lived only at Woolwich. Among the towns close to Dagenham, Barking and Romford recorded 200 and 109 plague deaths respectively during 1665, and places in the west of the county and in Hertfordshire also registered deaths from the disease, including Epping, Waltham Abbey, Hertford, Ware and St Albans.[12]

In the north of Essex, Ralph Josselin, the vicar of Earls Colne, ten miles from Colchester, was very aware of the progress of the plague in London and the risk that it posed to his own area. He noted the figures from the *Bills of Mortality* and the steady increase in the number of victims during the summer of 1665, anxious in case the disease appeared in nearby towns. Early in August his fears were realised when it was identified at Colchester, the culprit being a joiner who then moved on to Dedham, where he was incarcerated in the pest-house. Then plague was reported in Harwich, Ipswich, Braintree and Kelvedon, and Josselin was apprehensive that it would reach Coggeshall and indeed had begun already at Halstead, just three miles away. This was a confusing time for Josselin, who regarded the 'hand of god which is lifted up' as the cause of the outbreak, for although he saw little sign of the repentance that surely was demanded, his own village of 'sinful Colne' was spared, and God sent favourable weather for both a good harvest and the autumn sowing. An alarm came in the following spring when a woman died and plague was suspected as the cause, and so Josselin 'procured her speedie buriall'.[13] He was not alone in his anxiety. At Wimbish, near Saffron Walden, the recipe for an 'antipestilential preservative' was copied into the parish register itself.[14]

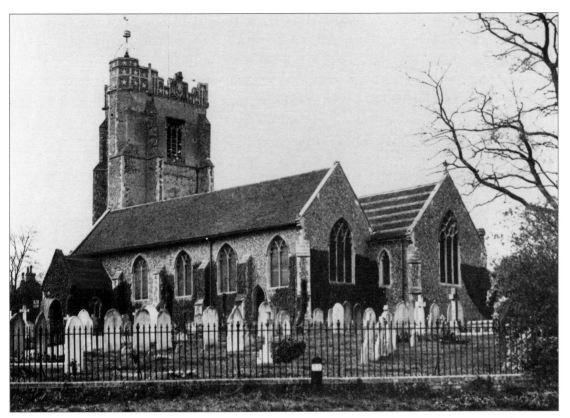

St Andrew's, Earls Colne, Essex. Ralph Josselin, the parson, anxiously checked the spread of the plague through the county. (© Crown copyright, NMR)

Despite such understandable concern, generally the rural communities in Essex escaped lightly, except for those that were at risk of infection from nearby towns, such as Moulsham near Chelmsford and Great Oakley, close to Harwich. At Great Oakley there were thirty-four deaths, twenty-three of them attributed to plague, between August and December 1666. Roughly 10 per cent of the inhabitants died during this period, and about 20 per cent of households were affected. Not all of the families who suffered a loss could be classified as poor, for the epidemic also struck those in the yeomen and husbandmen groups. At least one of the practices followed in urban communities was also observed in this village, for most of the plague victims were buried at night. Interments in unconsecrated ground were mentioned when the plague struck some rural areas. At Aldham, a few miles from Colchester, several plague deaths were recorded in

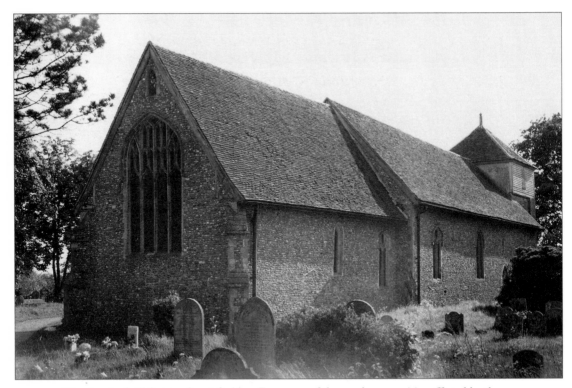

The church of All Saints, Great Oakley, Essex, one of the rural communities affected by the plague. (© Crown copyright, NMR)

1666, with one of the bodies interred in an orchard. More seriously, from the point of view of common decency as well as the risk to health, the body of Widow Foster of Danbury was left 'almost three days in the yard at the mercy of hogs and dogs'. She had died of plague while serving as a nurse to a family who claimed to have been suffering from nothing worse than 'a common ague and a fever'.[15]

The experience of many towns in Essex and Suffolk contrasted with that of the rural communities, with a number of them recording high levels of mortality. Some found the maintenance of their precautionary measures complicated by the presence of Dutch prisoners of war, their guards and wounded English seamen. Both coastal and inland towns were used to quarter the prisoners and wounded, including Colchester, Ipswich, Woodbridge, Hadleigh and Sudbury. More than 1,100 prisoners were lodged in the church at Sudbury, guarded by four companies of foot soldiers, for at least eight months. The malodorous conditions in the building were recognised to be 'dangerous for infection'. At Colchester more than

2,000 prisoners, with their guards, were held at the end of June, and by early August Ipswich contained two companies of foot soldiers, 1,600 sick and wounded seamen from the fleet, and 300 Dutch prisoners. The number of prisoners was later reduced as they were dispersed among other towns, but there were still 349 prisoners at Colchester and 59 at Ipswich in mid-November. The death of several of the 150 prisoners incarcerated at Hadleigh caused alarm, although inspection of the corpses showed that they had not died of plague.[16]

Colchester was a large and wealthy town with a population perhaps as high as 11,000, including an immigrant Dutch community that may have numbered 1,500, and the proportion of households exempt from paying the hearth tax was 52 per cent. The textile industry dominated the local economy, involving 40 per cent of the workforce, with weavers and the makers of bays and says, the 'new draperies', the most numerous occupations. The town was also a considerable port, with overseas as well as coastal trading links, exporting a range of commodities in addition to textiles, and importing coal, wine and a variety of manufactured goods and foodstuffs. This function made it more vulnerable to plague than the inland towns in the county, and it carried on a substantial trade with Rotterdam, where the disease had struck in 1664.[17] Furthermore, the precautions taken by the corporation to safeguard the town as plague began to erupt elsewhere in East Anglia in 1665 were put at risk when the prisoners and their guards were held there after the battle of Lowestoft in June.[18]

The outbreak was not attributed to the coming of the prisoners to the town, however, and indeed began a few weeks later. Josselin was aware of it by 13 August and a week later noted that Colchester's inhabitants 'seeke into the country for dwellings'. Before the end of September the merchant Nicholas Corsellis had moved away and reported that trade between Colchester and Ostend had been suspended because of the plague.[19] The corporation was quick to appoint bearers of the dead and searchers, who were enjoined to stay away from their families and to avoid other company, carrying white wands and keeping 'as far distant from men as may be'. The bearers were to carry out all burials during the night, unless ordered otherwise. Other measures taken during the epidemic were the conventional ones, such as marking infected houses with crosses, constructing two pest-houses and appointing a man to kill dogs and cats. Assistance for those who were infected and the poor who were thrown out of work became a major problem for the corporation. In October 1665 Josselin put the cost at £500 per month. The maintenance of the Dutch prisoners was also an expensive operation. Collections within Colchester proved to be inadequate and

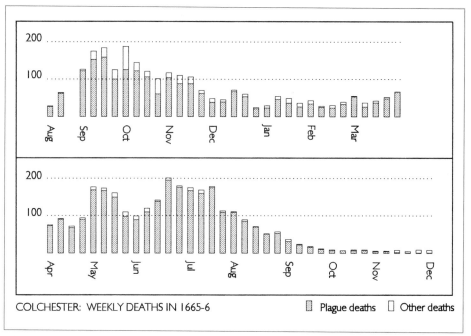

The numbers of deaths and plague-deaths in Colchester, August 1665–December 1666.
(© Michael Clements)

so a rate was levied on parishes within five miles of the town, and the area was later extended to cover part of the county. In addition, various charitable donations totalling £270 were received, and in May 1666 collections were taken in London churches which raised almost half the total receipts of just over £2,700. This seems to have been adequate, for a surplus of £81 remained at the end of April 1667.[20]

The number of deaths in Colchester rose sharply during August and September 1665, from 28 in the week ending 21 August to 126 during the first week in September and 184 a fortnight later.[21] A fall of 59 in the following week was welcomed by Josselin, but the next *Bill* showed a rise again, to 188 deaths in the week ending 6 October. This proved to be the peak for 1665 and the numbers declined steadily during the autumn, with the exception of an increase during one week, yet rose during the middle two weeks of December, as they did in London. Not until the end of the year did the number fall to that recorded in the middle of August. The winter saw fluctuating numbers of deaths, but those attributed to plague continued to form a high proportion of the total. Indeed, during

September, October and November plague deaths were 85 per cent of the total, and from the beginning of December until the end of March 1666 they were 86 per cent.

Josselin associated cold, frosty weather with a decline in the plague, commenting in December 'god purge our aire and heale the nation', and at the beginning of February that there were cold winds, frost and snow 'purging the aire, plague abates'. Yet the figures for Colchester show that at the end of February and into March the death toll rose once more. By March almost one in eight houses in the town stood empty because of deaths and departures.[22] Following a steady increase in deaths during the spring, the number reached 177 in the week ending 4 May, the first of two peaks during 1666. The second came in the third week of June, when 201 deaths were recorded. In July Pepys noted that the epidemic was so severe and prolonged that it was thought that it 'will quite depopulate the place'. Not until early October were the weekly numbers of deaths in single figures. During the period from April to the end of September 1666 plague deaths were almost 96 per cent of the total. This suggests that the practice of concealing plague deaths under other causes, which was commented on at

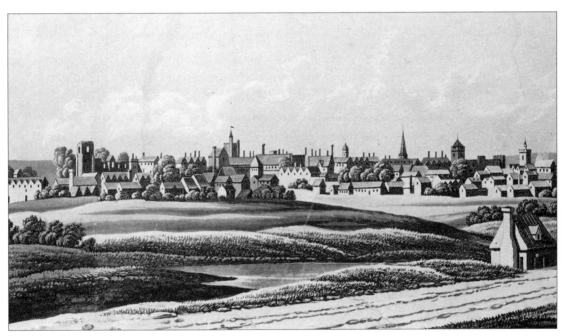

A view of Colchester, published in Cosimo, Duke of Tuscany's account of his visit to England, 1669. (© Colchester Library)

London, can hardly have been carried out in Colchester. Figures compiled by the eighteenth-century clergyman and historian Philip Morant give a total of 5,345 deaths between 14 August 1665 and 14 December 1666, of which 4,817, or 90 per cent, were attributed to plague. Thus, roughly a half of the population of the town died during the period, although it had been swollen for a time by the influx of soldiers and prisoners. The scale of the mortality and temporary absence of those who were able to get away is reflected in the low numbers of deaths late in 1666, with a weekly average of just over seven deaths from all causes during October and November.[23]

The chronology of the epidemic at Colchester showed a distinctly different pattern of deaths from that in London, where the plague continued to claim victims during 1666, but far fewer than in the previous year, and with no marked intensification. Generally, the pattern in the provinces was that the number of deaths from plague decreased during the winter, before increasing to epidemic levels again in 1666. The winter months were not unusually mild, nor was the period March to May 1666 especially warm, in the context of the 1660s. But the ensuing summer was a hot one, with a mean temperature considerably higher than that for any year since 1659, and both July and August were warmer than any of the corresponding months during the decade. A further distinctive feature of the weather was that both 1665 and 1666 were unusually dry years and included a long drought in south-east England that lasted from November 1665 until the following September.[24]

Mortality at Harwich and Ipswich followed this pattern, with epidemic conditions in both years. The outbreak at Harwich in the summer and autumn of 1665 claimed 100 victims in three weeks in September and early October, out of 414 deaths during the year, and the churchyard was said to be full. Further deaths from plague were reported as late as the middle of October 1666.[25] The corporation at Ipswich adopted standard measures against the plague in 1665, controlling entry to the town and prohibiting strangers without health certificates. But the numbers of burials began to increase during May and, although it was reported to be healthy in July, there was an alarm when William Huggard, a surgeon and controller of the customs, pronounced that the deaths of two people had been caused by plague. Huggard's diagnosis was not only not accepted by two surgeons sent to give their opinions, but was attributed to his personal hostility to the members of the corporation. By early August conditions in the town had become more difficult, with the presence of soldiers, prisoners, sick and wounded, and plague erupted soon afterwards. Whatever the origin of the outbreak, in September, October and November more deaths were recorded than in any other months during the century, with 662 in nine of the twelve parishes. Josselin noted that the plague was 'hott' in the town early in October, the peak month, but it did not attract his attention again, despite a resurgence of the disease in 1666, when the number of deaths peaked in July and August. The corporation took steps to contain the outbreak, by banning the markets and fairs and reducing the number of weekly lectures from two to one. Its efforts to provide for the poor were hampered because receipts from the rates were reduced due to the absence of many of the citizens, with 109 of the 2,000 houses standing empty. Between May 1665 and October 1666 there were 1,248 burials in the nine parishes for which the records survive, suggesting a total of at least 1,600, the equivalent of roughly 17 per cent of the population.[26]

Among the smaller East Anglian towns which suffered severely in the outbreak were the textile centres of Bocking and Braintree, standing close together in the middle of Essex. Bocking contained 361 households in 1670 and so probably had a population of no more than 1,800 before the outbreak. By May 1665 the plague was already so well established that the inhabitants were unclear who was 'safe' and free from the disease. During 1665 and 1666 the plague claimed 441 victims, and the total number of burials represented a crisis mortality ratio of 7.8. Braintree was slightly smaller, with 286 households, no fewer than 221 of which became infected. Between 5 September 1665 and 15 September 1666 there were 665 deaths from plague and another 22 of the inhabitants contracted the disease but survived, a mortality rate of almost 97 per cent. In 36 per cent of the infected households there was only one death, in 26 per cent there were two and in 19 per cent there were three. More than three deaths occurred in 19 per cent of the households in which plague fatalities were recorded. The number of deaths noted at Braintree may be too low, however, as the disease had struck Bocking in May and it is possible that it had spread to its neighbour before September. Even so, the available data suggest that roughly half the population of Braintree died in the epidemic, and a quarter of that of Bocking. Both towns were relatively poor. In 1670 as many as 81 per cent of householders at Bocking were exempt from paying the hearth tax because of poverty, and at Braintree the proportion was 66 per cent. During the epidemic Braintree received help from the surrounding area not only by collections, to distribute to the poor and provide the funds to pay for a physician and an apothecary, but also with the donation of two bullocks each week while the epidemic continued and thirty sheep.[27]

Just seven miles from Braintree and lying on the main road from Chelmsford to Colchester, Witham would seem to have been particularly vulnerable. Yet the only increase in burials during the plague years was a modest one in August and September 1666, and none of the deaths were noted as being from plague. Woodbridge, on the River Deben, suffered much greater mortality, with 300 deaths recorded in 1666, representing perhaps 25 per cent of the population, and at Framlingham there were 111 burials between July and October in the same year. The plague also struck Needham Market, eight miles from Ipswich, although Stowmarket, a further four miles inland, was not affected, nor was Lowestoft, despite its vulnerability as a port.[28]

Great Yarmouth was both larger than Lowestoft and had wider trading links, including connections with the United Provinces and Hamburg. It had been an early victim in 1602, when the plague had broken out in the town a year before the epidemic began in London and Norwich, and the same pattern occurred again in the 1660s, with cases recorded there in November 1664. The outbreak was blamed on a vessel trading with Rotterdam and continued throughout the winter and into 1665. By May the county justices had attempted to seal off the town, placing guards to prevent the citizens leaving and the country people from entering. The topography allowed the cordon to be held so effectively that those remaining became short of provisions. Josselin commented on the outbreak at Yarmouth before the end of May and a physician and surgeon to the pest-houses had been appointed by 9 June, when an apothecary was ordered to supply medicines 'to persons infected within this towne'. The reluctance of the inhabitants to undergo the expense of building 'cleansing houses' was blamed for the spread of the disease, which claimed an ever-increasing number of victims during July and August.

The heaviest weekly mortality came in late August and early September. During the last two weeks of August, 237 deaths were reported, 196 of them attributed to plague, and the total burials in the first week of September reached 139, with almost 500 during the month. The number of burials fell thereafter, but the epidemic continued until the following March, with a few intermittent deaths from plague until October, and claimed perhaps as many as 1,780 victims, from a population of roughly 10,000 before the onset of the disease. Those who died included the parish clerk, two apothecaries, two surgeons and the curate, Lionel Gadford, while some of the wealthier citizens moved away, to the irritation of the poor, 'being deprived of the charity and trade of the inhabitants, who are fled'. Those who left included members of the common council, so many of whom moved out of the town, or were unwilling to attend a meeting, that over a fourteen-month period during the outbreak six attempts to hold a sitting failed because not enough councillors appeared to constitute a quorum.[29]

The outbreak naturally caused anxiety at Norwich, which had a considerable trade through Yarmouth. Norwich was the largest provincial city in the seventeenth century, with a population of more than 20,000 in the 1660s, and it had a variety of roles. It was the seat of a diocese, a market centre of regional importance for grain and livestock, especially cattle, much of which was moved to London, and it contained an important textile industry producing the 'new draperies'. Of those admitted to the freedom of the city in the 1660s, 41 per cent were engaged in the textile trades, and by far the majority of them were worsted weavers. But a further characteristic of the city was the level of poverty among the population, with 62 per cent of householders exempt from paying the hearth tax.

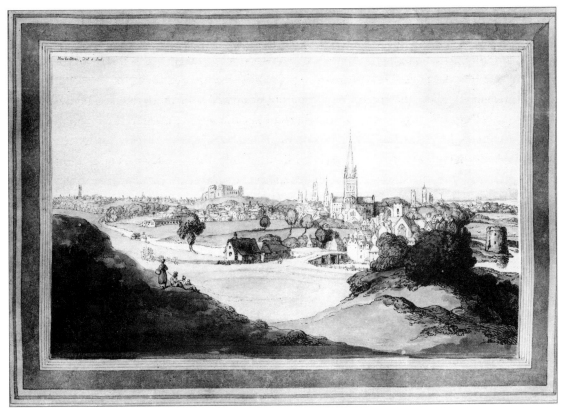

Norwich, 'a city in an orchard'. (© Crown copyright, NMR)

This unusually high ratio may have been partly because weavers' and dyers' furnaces were classified as exempt, but, even so, the figures suggest a considerable proportion of poor in the population, as in the other textile towns of East Anglia. In contemporaries' eyes this made it vulnerable to plague. On the other hand, the amount of space within the built-up area that was given over to gardens and orchards was commented on favourably by several visitors, including Thomas Fuller, who thought that it could be seen as either 'a city in an orchard or an orchard in a city', while John Evelyn noticed the flower gardens 'which all the inhabitants excell in' and found 'the prospect sweete'.[30]

A feature of Norwich which should have helped the authorities to prevent an outbreak of plague was the large proportion of the population living inside the city walls. As late as 1690, nine-tenths of its citizens were within the intramural area. Vetting of travellers arriving from elsewhere was far easier in those towns which were still encircled by walls, with the limited points of access through their gates, than in the unwalled ones. Nevertheless, Norwich had suffered from several outbreaks of plague in the late sixteenth and early seventeenth centuries, most severely in 1579, with a crisis mortality ratio of 12.3, and in 1603–4 and 1625–6. Both 1603 and 1625 had been years of heavy plague mortality in London, and epidemics there, where Norwich's cloth was marketed, and at Yarmouth prompted the city's authorities to take precautions.[31]

Following the outbreak of plague in 1664, vessels coming from Yarmouth to Norwich were stopped outside the city and their cargoes taken out to air before they could be admitted. The measures which were taken seem to have been successful during the summer of 1665, but by September plague had appeared in the city. In that month the danger was such that the city's most distinguished citizen, Sir Thomas Browne, physician and author of *Religio Medici*, left, together with his family. There were nineteen plague deaths in the last week of October, but although the disease was present during the following winter and spring, it attracted little attention.[32]

The early summer of 1666 brought an increase in the number of deaths from the contagion and the scale of the growing problem had become apparent by early July, when the town clerk, Thomas Corie, wrote that 'The plague grows fast amongst us: and poverty faster.'[33] The cost and administration of the relief for the rising numbers of poor during the epidemic was a great concern to Corie, who returned to the theme in several letters to Joseph Williamson, and visited London to petition the king for assistance. His management of the crisis was not helped by the fact that many of the aldermen left – part of a general exodus of 'the men of best estates'. It was estimated that by the third week of July a quarter of the citizens would have departed, at a time when, as Corie reported, 'The plague encreaseth dayly' and the poor were becoming so resentful that they were threatening to occupy the houses that had been left empty. Both the total numbers of deaths and those attributed to plague rose steadily throughout July and by the end of the month no parish was free from the disease, which had also been reported in some villages. Even so, an attempt to move the market out of the city to a site half a mile away was ignored.[34]

After a hopeful return for the first week in August that showed a slight decrease in deaths, the numbers again increased, until the week of 15–22 August in which 220 died, 203 of them from plague. This was the worst week, and the numbers declined thereafter, albeit slowly and erratically, with 574 burials in September, compared with 498 in July. By mid-September Corie admitted that 'Wee are in greater feare of the poore than the plague, all our monie being gone', for he had earlier pointed out that it was money that kept them in check and that when no more was available for relief 'we feare they will be unrulie'. The weekly

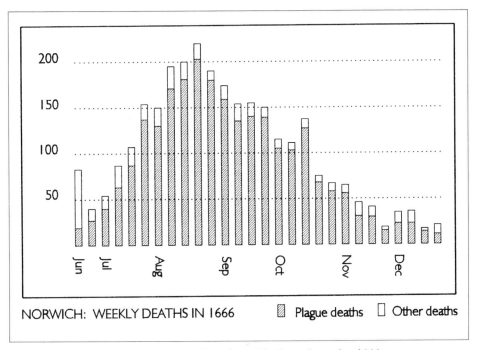

NORWICH: WEEKLY DEATHS IN 1666   ▨ Plague deaths ▢ Other deaths

The numbers of deaths and plague-deaths in Norwich, June–December 1666.
(© Michael Clements)

cost was almost £250, and when he wrote to Williamson on 19 September he had received the alarming news that there had been an increase in the number of deaths in the previous week, with thirty further houses infected. Even after falls over the next fortnight, another sharp rise in the numbers followed. Only with the cooler weather and a further decline in the numbers of plague deaths could he be sure that the epidemic was on the wane. His anxieties regarding the poor were alleviated by a timely bumper catch of herring by the Yarmouth fishermen, and so he could turn his attention away from the consequences of the epidemic to the threat posed by the nonconformists. The winter did not bring a complete end to the outbreak, however, for further deaths from the disease were reported in the spring of 1667, with the last being registered in early June.[35]

The total number of burials recorded in Norwich between 3 October 1665 and 26 December 1666 was 3,682, with 2,810 of the deaths attributed to plague. Other deaths during the outbreak occurred both before and after this period; allowing for these, it seems that almost 20 per cent of the city's population died during the epidemic. The proportion of deaths from plague was at its highest during the summer of 1666, accounting for 93.5 per cent of the total of 2,032 between 20 June and 3 October.[36] The greatest levels of mortality were in the poorest districts, especially among the inhabitants of those parishes on low-lying land to the south of the city centre and in the parish of St James on the north side of the River Wensum. The mortality rate in the poor parishes was three times that of the prosperous central ones, and the geography of the plague broadly reflected the distribution of wealth, for the poor districts suffering high numbers of deaths were those which lay around an affluent core, where the epidemic had much less impact.[37]

In the western part of East Anglia, plague struck at towns on the network of waterways that drained into the Wash, including King's Lynn, Ely, Peterborough, Ramsey and Cambridge. King's Lynn escaped relatively lightly, with the modest total of twenty-two deaths from the disease between late August and early November 1665, as did Ely, which was described as infected, yet experienced higher numbers of deaths in 1667–8 and 1680. The other three towns were affected more seriously. Although it lay some distance from the main roads, the risk of the contagion at Ramsey may have been increased by its riverborne trade. Much of the town's importance derived from Ramsey Lode, a channel connecting the town directly to the River Nene, an important waterway which also carried 'Boats, barges and vessels of large size . . . from the ports of Wisbich and Lynn, to the . . . city of Peterborough.' The 400 deaths during an outbreak in 1666 comprised roughly 30 per cent of the population, and the plague also affected the nearby villages of Coppingford and Upton.[38] The epidemic was of much longer duration at Peterborough, beginning in the summer of 1665 and continuing until May 1667, with approximately 470 deaths, 351 of them attributed to plague. Roughly 17 per cent of the town's population died during this period. Only a few of the victims of the disease were buried in the churchyard, most of the remainder being interred at the pest-house, and forty-seven of them in gardens, orchards or other ground attached to the deceased's property.[39]

At Cambridge there were 413 burials in 1665 and 797 in 1666, together about 15 per cent of the population of almost 8,000.[40] The university dispersed in the summer of 1665, gradually reassembled in the following spring, but when the number of plague deaths again rose, it was dismissed on 22 June. The scholars were not permitted to return before January 1667. Their absence, together with that of many of the senior members, contributed significantly to the disruption of the town's economy, as did the cancellation of Stourbridge fair. Although the weekly *Bills* for the town carried the notice that all of the colleges were free from the disease, in fact the manciple of Christ's died of plague, with the result that 'all fled from the Colledge', and in October 1665 those remaining at Clare were 'all lockt in', the master not even entrusting the porter with the keys. Partly because those who stayed took such care to preserve their isolation, and partly because of their ability to move away, the members of the university largely escaped. The wealthier citizens, too, were able to leave. Alderman Samuel Newton's family moved to Waterbeach on 23 June 1666 and returned on 26 October. As elsewhere, the poorer citizens of the town were the most vulnerable to the disease.[41]

The towns along the Thames downstream from London and those on the Medway were as exposed as the ports and textile towns in East Anglia, from their contact with the capital and involvement in coastal and overseas trade. The intensification of naval activity during the war with the Dutch increased the risk, by bringing overcrowding to the dockyard towns and by the landing of prisoners and sick and wounded seamen who were infected. Evelyn reported in February 1666 that eighty-four of the sailors put ashore at nine ports in Kent over the previous fifteen months had died of plague. In mid-August 1665 Pepys noted that the plague was 'great' in Gravesend, and before the end of the month that it had begun 'to grow very great' at Greenwich, Woolwich and Deptford. These were communities which had experienced rapid growth during the seventeenth century, with the associated problems of uncontrolled building and social dislocation. In 1659 Deptford had been described as consisting largely of small tenements, recently built.[42]

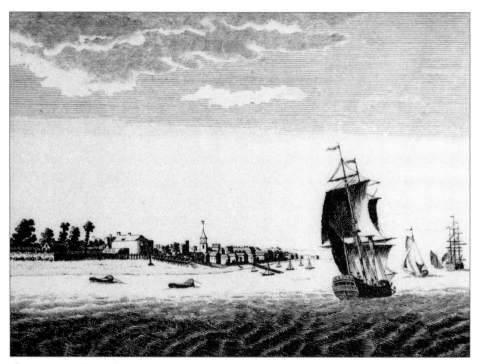

Gravesend in 1775. (© Crown copyright, NMR)

Plague had begun to be such a threat in Deptford by the last week in August 1665 that John Evelyn sent his wife and most of his household to his brother's house at Wotton, although he felt that his duties prevented him from leaving. On 9 September he mentioned that almost thirty houses were infected, and by the end of the month he was seriously alarmed, writing that he and Sir William Doyly, who were Commissioners for the Sick and Wounded, were 'at every moment at the mercy of a raging pestilence'. The situation was no better in mid-October, when Evelyn reported that he felt 'in perpetual danger . . . there is almost no house cleere'. No respite came in 1666, and in July the inhabitants claimed that the plague 'rageth at present more sorely than ever'. The burial figures support their statement, for 374 deaths were attributed to plague during 1665, but 522 were similarly classified in 1666. Gravesend, too, was 'very much infected' in 1666, as it had been in 1665, with 352 burials in the twelve months following September 1665. This followed a ten-year period of unusually low mortality, during which the annual number of burials fluctuated between twenty and forty.[43]

Even in these towns close to the capital, the chronology of the epidemic was different from that in London, with the death toll rising as high, or higher, in 1666 as it had done in 1665. The date at which the epidemic began also differed, both from its onset in London, and in towns that lay relatively close together. The first plague burial in Chatham took place on 20 August 1665, in Sittingbourne on 14 September, yet in Gillingham not until 7 October. At Chatham the disease was prevalent by early October, making less impact during the winter, but increasing again in the summer of 1666, with up to nine burials in a day being reported, and 100 houses infected in early August. It continued to claim victims in the town in 1667, for there were seven plague deaths in July and August. Rochester, Deal, Sandwich and Dover were also badly affected by the epidemic. At Rochester, 500 burials were recorded between April and December 1665, from a population of perhaps 3,000. In August 1666 the corporation appealed for help because the epidemic had lasted for over a year and still continued. Plague was reported at Dover in August 1665, and as late as October 1666 deaths were still occurring at a rate of forty or fifty a week. In all, there were at least 900 plague deaths in the town, which lost between one-quarter and one-third of its population. An even higher estimate for Deal put the loss at three-quarters of those who had remained, which may indicate that a large number of citizens had left to avoid the disease, as well as a very high level of mortality. In August 1666 Evelyn told Pepys that 'the towne is almost quite depopulated'. The inland towns of Canterbury and Maidstone appear to have suffered less heavily during the epidemic. The appearance of the disease at Canterbury in November was blamed on the greed of the two victims, one of whom had gone to London and returned with goods from towns where the plague was known to be present, and the other had sent for goods from infected places. Maidstone was the cause of an alarm in August 1667, when the disease was said to have broken out 'with great violence' and spread among many houses because the magistrates had neglected to take effective action. This was among the last outbreaks of the epidemic.[44]

In Kent, as elsewhere, it was the densely populated urban parishes which suffered most deaths. Rural communities were less likely to be infected, and those which did contain plague victims were scattered. Only 14 per cent of a sample of communities in Kent had crisis mortality ratios of more than 1.5 in 1665 and 1666. For East Sussex the proportion was slightly higher, 16 per cent of the sample in 1665 and 21 per cent in 1666. But these increases in mortality were from all deaths and not caused solely by plague. Nevertheless, the disease lingered

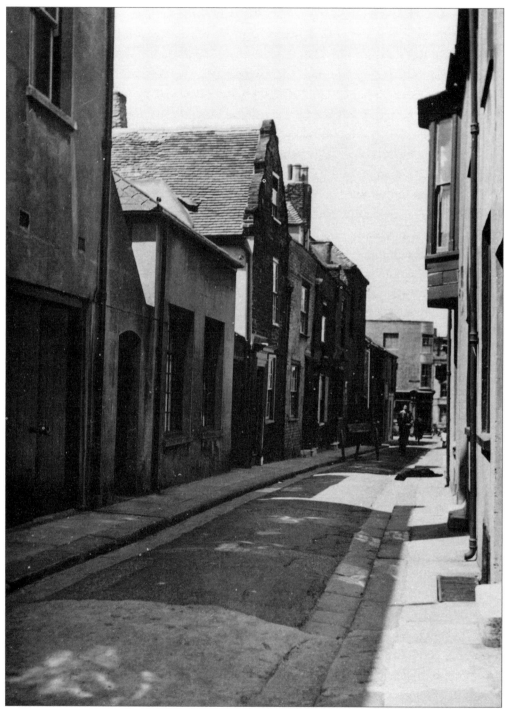

Dolphin Street, Deal, in 1947. The town was badly affected by the plague in 1666. (© Crown copyright, NMR)

on in the Weald into the late 1660s, with twelve plague deaths at Biddenden in 1667, where twelve others contracted plague but recovered, and six deaths from 'the sickness' at Pembury in May 1668.[45]

Plague may have made an early appearance in the Hampshire towns at Fareham, where the number of burials began to rise in May 1665, continuing at an abnormally high level during June and into early July. The disease continued to claim victims there until September 1666, but the pattern was erratic, with an increase in burials during the winter, in November and December, and January having the highest monthly total recorded. A little over half the deaths occurred between November 1665 and the following April, although there was a further peak in July and August. The total number of burials in 1665 was 56 and in the following year 79, the highest numbers for any year since the plague of 1563, when there had been 83 burials. A feature of the epidemic in 1665–6 was that it was widely spread among the families in the town, with 60 per cent or more of them losing at least one member. Similarly, at Petersfield 45 per cent of the 112 affected families lost just one member, and a further 25 per cent lost two. Perhaps 20 per cent of the town's population died in 1666, with a total of 254 burials, representing a crisis mortality ratio of 11.0. The pattern of deaths shows a steady rise from the first plague burial on 5 April to a single peak, in the week ending 3 July, with a high level of mortality during July and a decline thereafter. The recorded plague deaths occurred in a period of twenty-eight weeks, between April and October. By the end of 1665 the disease had been identified at Kingsclere, in the north of the county. Houses of suspected victims were shut up and guarded, and the occupants were kept supplied with provisions. Some families were moved to an area of wasteland near the town, where burials of some plague victims took place and perhaps where the new pest-house was erected. Those suffering from plague were treated with 'cordiales and plague water and medicaments for theire smoking', as well as ointments, angelica water and treacle. The sums paid by the churchwardens and overseers in 1665-6 were £110 5s 3d, but this was only 36 per cent higher than their outgoings for the previous year. Contributions from the surrounding area and a donation of £20 from George Morley, Bishop of Winchester, together with the parish rate, were more than enough to cover their total expenditure.[46]

Southampton suffered badly during the second half of 1665 and throughout much of 1666. The plague was identified there in June 1665 and by early July things were so bad that the mayor appealed to the Privy Council for aid. In late September Thomas Rugg noted that the mortality was as serious as in London, in

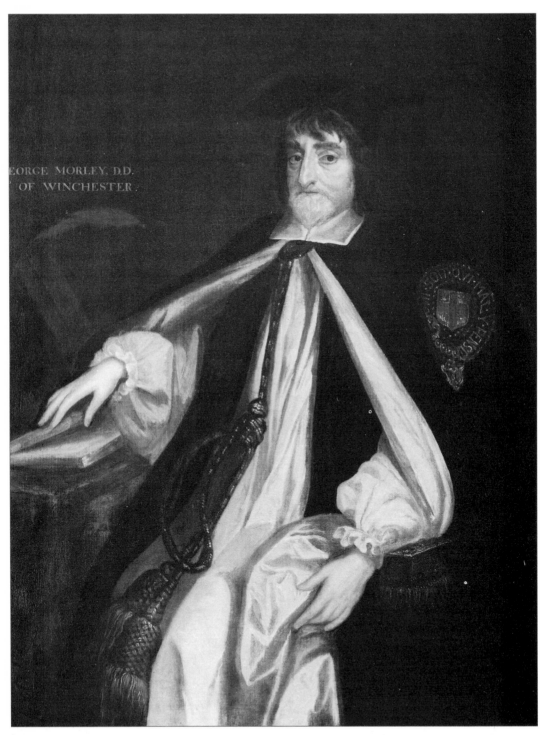

George Morley, Bishop of Winchester 1662–84, after Sir Peter Lely. (© Crown copyright, NMR)

proportion to the population. Indeed, it seems to have been far worse, for in 1683 the corporation put the number of dead at 1,700. Even allowing for some exaggeration in their letter, in which they pleaded for especial consideration because of the town's poverty, this suggests a high percentage of deaths in a population of rather more than 3,000, and a level of mortality on a par with that at Colchester. The scale of the epidemic was such that it produced a breakdown in parochial registration, the removal of the wealthier citizens, parish clergy and officers, and fears of social disorder because of the inability of the authorities to provide relief for the poor. Because the clergy had left, the French pastor undertook the baptism of infants and conducted a marriage. He wrote that the disease had compelled 'most people' to leave their houses. The corporation later took action against those in responsible positions who had fled, fining the deputy mayor and sixteen officers for being absent during the crisis.[47]

Other Hampshire towns escaped the plague in 1665, only to suffer in 1666, including Basingstoke, Portsmouth and Winchester. There had been great concern at Portsmouth during 1665 because of the overcrowded conditions, exacerbated by the war with the Dutch. The dangers were increased by seamen and their families travelling there from London and carpenters coming from Southampton to work in the dockyard, when both areas were experiencing epidemics. The magistrates took action against householders who had lodged travellers from those places, and despite the danger, the measures which they implemented seem to have been successful, for no deaths from plague were recorded until January 1666.[48] But when the disease did strike, the conditions produced similar problems to those reported in Southampton, with disruption of the markets and consequent shortage of provisions, inadequate space in the pest-house and the added difficulty of trying to keep the dockyard free from the disease. Carpenters who had been in infected houses were ordered to wash themselves and their clothes, and burn resin and brimstone for fourteen days before they could be allowed into the yard. Provocative antisocial behaviour was also reported, with Thomas Middleton, the Navy Commissioner, informing Pepys that plague victims were taking the 'foul plasters from their sores' and throwing them into the windows of uninfected houses at night. William Smegergill told Pepys of similar behaviour in Westminster, where 'bold people' would lean out of their windows and breathe in the faces of passers-by. In neither case did Pepys's informant claim to be an eyewitness, and such reports may be typical of stories, with a strong social bias, born of the fear that was prevalent in such dangerous times. The tensions in Portsmouth did lead to disorder, however, with some of those confined to their houses breaking out 'to visitt the houses of the better sort' and releasing the prisoners from the gaol. The trained bands dispersed the crowd, but only by using violence, killing one man and wounding three others. During 1666 there were 436 burials in Portsmouth, a crisis mortality ratio of more than 3.5, with 187 attributed to plague between April and August. Mortality remained high in 1667, which saw 322 burials, but plague was not among the causes. Middleton reported 'fevers and distempers' in March, when more people were dying than during the plague epidemic.[49]

The cathedral cities of Winchester and Salisbury had similar experiences during the Great Plague. Precautions taken at Winchester in 1665 included the

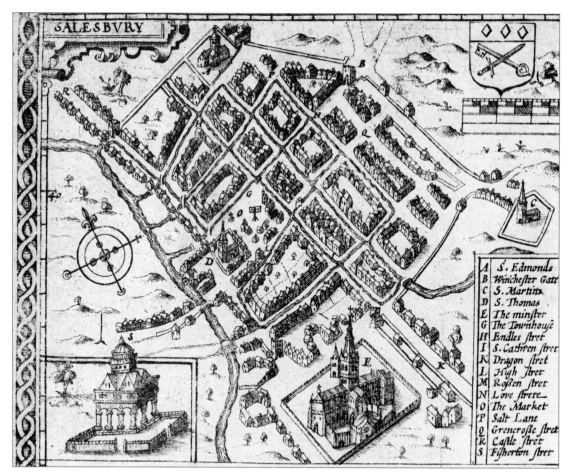

A	S. Edmonds
B	Winchester Gate
C	S. Martins
D	S. Thomas
E	The minster
G	The Townhouse
H	Endles stret
I	S. Cathren stret
K	Dragon stret
L	High stret
M	Rossen stret
N	Love strete
O	The Market
P	Salt Lane
Q	Grencroste stret
R	Castle stret
S	Fisherton stret

After leaving Hampton Court, the court took refuge at Salisbury, until cases of plague were reported in the city. (© Crown copyright, NMR)

control of entry to the city, the issue of orders 'for the more cleanlyness, decency and sweetness of the eyre' and the cancellation of the mayor's supper and other feasts in the autumn. Nevertheless, a serious epidemic in the following year brought the almost complete disruption of parish registration, the closure of Winchester College in August, the discontinuation of services in the cathedral, and an exodus of those who were able to leave. In June it was reported that 'All the town is emptied . . . into the country about' and in August conditions in the city were said to be 'as bad as evar considering the small nomber remaining in it'. The extent of the mortality is uncertain, but the outbreak was the worst in the city since 1625, and the corporation later claimed that 'many hundreds' had died. Although severe, the epidemic subsided quickly enough for the College to reopen on 1 December, although the quarter sessions were not held there again until the following April.[50]

Salisbury was chosen as a safe place for the court's sojourn after its withdrawal from London in July 1665. Despite concern that its presence would attract those with aspirations rather than genuine business, increasing the risk, controls were inadequate and by the beginning of August the city was 'encumbered with numbers of useless persons'.[51] Sure enough, plague was identified there during the month, and the court moved away in September. In fact, the disease made little impact in 1665, but in the following year it caused considerable disruption and perhaps more than 500 deaths, in a population of roughly 7,000. The epidemic prompted the comment that when plague was established in 'these little towns, it is more dangerous than in London itself, because less means of avoiding it'.[52]

Further west, deaths from plague occurred at Sherborne in November 1665 – the spread of the disease was attributed to people gathering at funerals – but the outbreak may not have been a severe one. In the following January the Wiltshire justices ordered a collection for the relief of the plague victims at Donhead St Mary, near Shaftesbury. They also issued general orders prohibiting tradesmen from receiving goods from places known to be infected, compelling those confined to their houses to remain in them, and restraining tinkers, pedlars and itinerant fiddlers from travelling around. Ogbourne St Andrew, Wootton Bassett, Marlborough and nearby Mildenhall, in the north of the county, were infected in 1666, but the disease seems to have made little impact in the West Country.[53] Just eight deaths were recorded in Plymouth in October 1666 and seventy-two at Bristol between April and September, in a city with a population approaching 20,000. The council at Bristol had acted promptly in 1665, setting watches in June to prevent anyone from London entering the city, although modifying this in the following February, when the watchmen were positioned not at the city's limits but at the gates into the intramural area. Indeed, most of the plague deaths occurred in the suburban parishes. In June 1666 the corporation claimed that the infection was confined to Bedminster, on the south side of the city, and those who were afflicted were being cared for in the pest-house.[54] Similar precautions were taken at Exeter, with watches set at the entrances to the town, people and goods from London prohibited from entering, the Magdalen and Lammas fairs cancelled and an order made for the completion of the pest-house. Evidently, these measures were successful, although one suspect from a town contaminated with plague did get into the city. The West Country ports as a whole escaped lightly, although potentially vulnerable to infection because of their seaborne trade.[55]

In the summer of 1666 two of Sir Heneage Finch's sons, who were studying at Oxford, were taken by their tutor on a tour to Bath, Wells, Bristol and Gloucester. It is improbable that they would have undertaken the journey had there been any risk from plague either at those cities or along their route.[56] The party did not venture as far up the Severn valley as Upton-upon-Severn, where there had been an outbreak in the previous year.[57] Further west, Hereford escaped and the death of Francis, Lord Vaughan, from plague at Ludlow Castle on 2 March 1667 seems to have been anomalous in both geographical and social terms. Indeed, while not immune, the Marches and Wales did not suffer heavily.[58] Chester was at risk because of its role as a port, especially for traffic with Ireland, but experienced only a minor outbreak and no apparent disruption.[59]

Following its departure from Salisbury, the court did not move further west, but to Oxford, which had been the royalist headquarters during the Civil War and was able to provide ample and appropriate accommodation in the colleges. Following the outbreak at Salisbury and the possibility that another move would be necessary if plague broke out, strong measures were taken. The university and the city justices combined to issue a set of 'Rules and Orders' and, based on the experience of overcrowding at Salisbury, a list of the inhabitants was compiled that distinguished inmates, so that those who were not residents, accredited members of the university or servants of courtiers could be expelled. This was the kind of procedure commonly followed in preparation for a siege, and was a particularly rigorous application of the steps taken to regulate a community during a plague epidemic. The royal guards were posted to control entry to the city, the university's officers being regarded as 'too weak'. Despite such care, one 'lewde fellow . . . haveinge a plague sore upon him' borrowed a scholar's gown and so managed to get in. When discovered he was

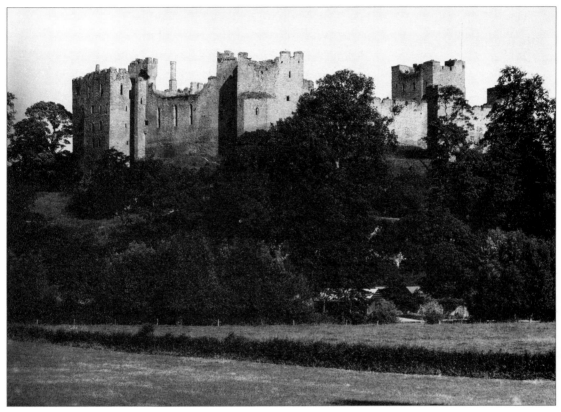

Francis Vaughan, Lord Vaughan, died from plague at Ludlow Castle in 1667. (© B.T. Batsford Ltd)

'dryven out agayne' and lodged in the pest-house, while two houses which he was known to have occupied were shut up. Movement of goods was also controlled. The mayor of Abingdon was instructed to prevent boats on the Thames from passing beyond the town until it had been ascertained that their cargoes had not come from a place where the disease had been identified. Even so, groceries and wines bought in the city were suspected of being brought covertly from London along the Thames. Although the regulations could not be completely maintained and there were fears of plague in the villages around, thought to have been transmitted by refugees from London, Oxford itself remained free of the disease. Parliament was able to meet in the city in October and the courts were adjourned there from Westminster, although those attending were required to produce health certificates.[60] This produced a considerable influx and overcrowding that increased the danger, yet the impression gained by one new arrival was that 'there is nothing here but mirth'.[61]

Reports of plague in the towns and villages between Oxford and London should have produced anxiety rather than mirth. Bruno Ryves felt distinctly unsafe in his rectory at Haseley, less than ten miles from Oxford, writing that 'we have been afraid one of another, as if the curse of Cain had been upon us, to fear that every man that met us would slay us . . . no man thought himself secure in his closest retirements'.[62] His fears would have been heightened by the appearance of plague even in a such a remote Chiltern village as Great Hampden. Places along the main lines of communication were more vulnerable, with the Thamesside towns of Windsor, Reading, Marlow and Wallingford all experiencing outbreaks of the disease. Windsor was unusually well prepared, however, for the pest-house had been repaired in 1659, because 'We know not how sone it maye pleasse God to send a visitacion'. The corporation's outlay of about £17 in preventive measures and relief during the Great Plague suggests that the town was not badly affected. Nor was Reading, where a rate was imposed to cover the cost of employing searchers and buriers, and for wardens to prevent the admittance of 'suspicious persons and goods'. The outbreaks in the towns on the Great West Road where the plague struck were 'not raging' and were short-lived. But some communities along the Thames did not escape so lightly, for the village of Little Marlow suffered fifty plague deaths in 1665.[63]

Away from the river, but on the route used by carriers plying between London and Oxford, 117 plague deaths were recorded at Uxbridge in 1665, and High Wycombe was badly affected in both 1665 and 1666, with two-thirds of the 293 burials during those years attributed to plague.[64] Despite eruptions such as these, the outbreak was not widespread. The aggregate number of burials for a sample of parishes across Berkshire shows no increase during the plague years. Indeed, the figures for those years were lower than for the early years of the decade.[65]

To the north-east of Oxford, in 1665 the small town of Bletchley, just off Watling Street, experienced a death rate six times its normal level, with 126 burials, and the increase in the number of deaths was even greater at Lavendon, between Bedford and Northampton.[66] Yet Northampton itself appears to have escaped, together with a number of other Midland towns, including Walsall, Leicester and Stafford, although the disease erupted in Lichfield, Coventry, Melton Mowbray, and in Newark-on-Trent, despite a report from the town in September 1665 that 'We keep strict watches here and hereabouts.'[67] William Hutton, the antiquarian, enthusiastically described the effects of destructive outbreaks at Birmingham and Derby, depicting Birmingham as 'depopulated' and Derby as 'forsaken'. Yet the evidence of the parish registers indicates that neither

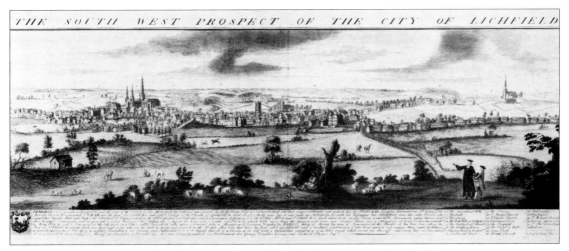

Lichfield, by Samuel and Nathaniel Buck, 1774. (© Crown copyright, NMR)

town suffered an epidemic of plague in 1665 or 1666. Higher than average mortality did occur at Birmingham in 1665–6, but came during the winter months and is unlikely to have been caused by plague, and the registers for Derby do not provide evidence of an upsurge in burials.[68] But Nottingham did experience an increase in deaths during 1667, which may indicate an outbreak of plague, with 219 burials, compared with 149 in 1665 and 180 in 1666.[69]

As elsewhere, urban communities in the Midlands were more likely to be affected by the plague than rural ones, but villages were by no means immune. Those that lay on the main roads, such as Meriden and Dunchurch in Warwickshire, were especially vulnerable.[70] Between 14 August and 17 October 1665, twenty-eight burials were recorded at Skeffington in Leicestershire, where the annual average was four. The villagers were said to have decamped to the woods to avoid the epidemic.[71] A completely different decision was taken by the inhabitants of Eyam, in northern Derbyshire, ten miles south-west of Sheffield. This large parish covered 3,000 acres, with the population distributed chiefly among three villages: Eyam itself, Grindleford Bridge and Foolow. The first casualty of the disease was George Vicars, a tailor, who died on 6 September 1665. Writing in 1744, Richard Mead attributed the origin of the epidemic at Eyam to clothes sent to Vicars from London in a chest and hung up to dry after being unpacked. According to his account, derived from the son of the rector during the epidemic, Vicars's wife was the only member of the household to survive. An alternative source of the infection that has been suggested was via visitors from

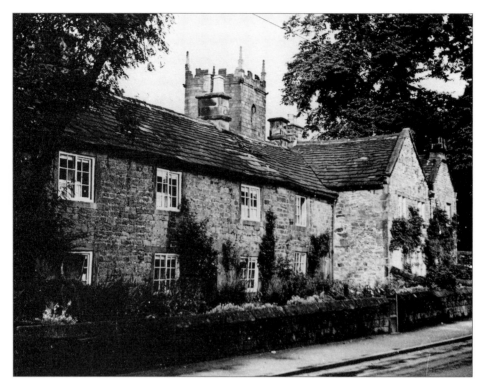

The plague cottages at Eyam, with St Lawrence's Church behind. (© Crown copyright, NMR)

Derby attending the Wakes – the annual commemoration of the dedication of the church – at Eyam on 20 August. This explanation seems to have been based on Hutton's misleading account of an epidemic at Derby in that summer. While the interval between the Wakes and Vicars's death provides plausibility for the suggestion, the absence of evidence for such an epidemic at Derby rather weakens it. Indeed, plague could have been brought to Eyam by any visitors to the Wakes, not just those from Derby.[72]

Following Vicars's death, there was an interval of fourteen days before the next burial, and there were just six interments in the parish during September. A sharp rise saw twenty-three burials in October, but there was then a decline during the winter and no appreciable increase until June 1666. From the start of November until the end of May there were thirty-three burials, roughly double the average for those months over the previous fifteen years. But June saw the beginnings of a much more severe outbreak, with twenty-one burials during the month. Afraid that his parishioners would take alarm and move away, spreading the disease around the neighbouring communities, the rector, William Mompesson, persuaded them not to leave, and his pleas were endorsed by his predecessor, Thomas Stanley. The common problem of providing support for sequestered victims was overcome when Mompesson obtained the promise of help from the Earl of Devonshire. Arrangements were made for the supply of provisions and huts were built for the sick. This selfless behaviour achieved the object of restricting the plague to Eyam, but the parish itself suffered a further 176 deaths between the beginning of July and the end of October, with 78 recorded in August, the worst month. In Mompesson's summary he reported that seventy-six families had been infected by plague, with a total of 259 deaths from the disease, while the entries in the parish register suggest that as many as eighty-nine families, or households, lost at least one member, and that the number of plague deaths was 260. A further sixteen deaths recorded during the epidemic presumably were from other causes. The whole parish had a population no lower than 850 and perhaps slightly more than 1,000, so that the 276 deaths during the fourteen months of epidemic represented between 27 and 32 per cent of the inhabitants. Eyam itself was the most populous of the three settlements in the parish and may have been the most heavily affected, with almost half its inhabitants dying. Indeed, Thomas Short, writing in 1749, reported that 'near half the People of the Village' had been casualties of the epidemic.[73]

Fewer than one-fifth of the families in Eyam who were affected were wiped out, and in slightly over one-fifth more both of the parents died. The most common outcome was that one of the married partners died, which occurred in half the families. Adults over twenty years old accounted for 54 per cent of the deaths during the fourteen months of the epidemic, the same proportion for that age group recorded over the previous fourteen years. But the pattern within the under-twenty age group changed significantly during the epidemic. In the pre-plague period infants and children under five years old accounted for 37 per cent of deaths, but during the epidemic this fell to 15 per cent, while the proportion of children aged five to ten rose from 3 per cent to 10 per cent of deaths and that of adolescents aged between ten and twenty increased even more, from 6 per cent to 20 per cent. Plague therefore brought a change in the age pattern of mortality, but it did not have an impact so far as gender was concerned, with 52 per cent of those who died being males, of all ages, only slightly smaller than the proportion recorded in non-plague years.[74]

Much less isolated than Eyam was Cawood, a village with a population of almost 1,000 on the Ouse ten miles south of York. It may have been vulnerable

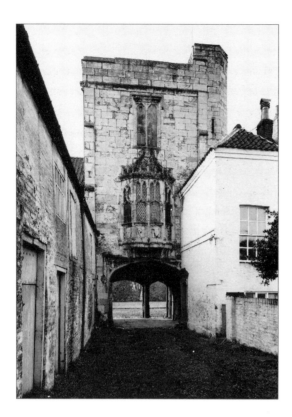

The gatehouse of Cawood Castle,
palace of the archbishops of York.
(© Crown copyright, NMR)

through its position on the river and because of the presence of the Archbishop of York's palace, which made it difficult to regulate the ingress of visitors. An outbreak there in 1500 had claimed the life of the Archbishop himself, Thomas Rotherham. The plague was identified on 21 July 1665 and by 9 September there had been roughly forty-five deaths, with nineteen houses closed. Within the next nine days there were another fifteen deaths, five on one day, and eleven more houses had been isolated, so that roughly one-sixth of those in the village were closed. By that stage of the epidemic two-thirds of the families were receiving relief and, equally seriously, few of the remainder were able to provide assistance. Through the influence of the archbishop, help was raised in York, but the rural communities in the area were not expected to be able to supply much aid.[75]

Poor relief was a problem faced by the members of the corporation at Newcastle upon Tyne. The expense during an outbreak of plague in 1665 was so high that, they claimed, the collections which were taken raised no more than one-tenth of the cost. The remainder was paid from the town's own coffers, and even after subsequent collections there was still a shortfall that amounted to 'a great deale of money'. In these circumstances the corporation was reluctant to hand over the sums collected to help the sufferers in Cambridge, preferring to use them to offset their own costs. The justices for County Durham had imposed a quarantine on shipping from London and Great Yarmouth as well as other measures, but not entirely successfully, for plague deaths were recorded at Sunderland, Gateshead and South Shields, as well as at Newcastle. Jeremy Reed, from Kent, was alleged to have been the 'bringer of the plague' to the region. He died on 5 July and the disease accounted for about thirty deaths in Sunderland in the following three months. Plague was identified again in Gateshead in January 1666 and the mayor of Newcastle reported that it was present in the autumn of that year and into the following winter.[76]

The Great Plague in the provinces began in 1664 and continued through into 1667, striking some communities in only one year, but others for a longer period, spanning two or, more rarely, three years. As with earlier plague epidemics, towns were more prone to an outbreak than were villages, with some of those attacked experiencing very high levels of mortality. Colchester, Braintree and Southampton may have lost half their inhabitants and in a number of other towns in East Anglia and southern England more than one-quarter of the inhabitants died. Yet the West Country and Wales were hardly affected, and the north-west, parts of the Midlands and much of the north of England largely escaped. Even within the regions most heavily visited, many communities had no deaths from the disease and no peak in the numbers of burials. Indeed, the epidemic was notable more for its intensity in the places that were affected than for its wide spread. But no clear pattern is discernible, for some communities escaped while others close by did not, and relatively remote places that were neither coastal nor inland ports and did not lie on any of the principal routes were infected. Neither remoteness nor the implementation of preventive policies and health measures provided certain protection from the plague bacillus, despite the steps taken by both borough and county justices, and the efforts of the parish officers. The outbreak was a perplexing problem, but one which stimulated activity and debate rather than fatalism and torpidity.

CHAPTER 4

Policy and Plague

The Plague was indeed an irreparable dammage to the whole Kingdom: but that which chiefly added to the misery, was the time, wherein it happen'd. For what could be a more deplorable accident, than that so many brave men should be cut off by the Arrow, that flies in the dark, when our Country was ingag'd in a foreign War, and when their Lives might have been honourably ventur'd on a glorious Theater in its defence?

Thomas Sprat, *The History of the Royal Society of London* (1667), p. 120

[Collections] for the succour of the miserably distressed in and about London and Westminster whose Calamity is farr more to be pityed than any elswhere, not only for the raging of the Infection, but even for the very want of Necessaries for life, Many perishing that way that otherwise might have bin recovered out of the danger, And many thowsands of poore Artisans being ready to starve for want of meanes to be imployed in their callings, all trading being become dangerous and layed aside by reason of the spreading of the Contagion.

Gilbert Sheldon to Humphrey Henchman, 31 July 1665

The government's preventive policies were put in place only when plague threatened, and others dealing with the effects of the disease once it had erupted. While Graunt's pioneering analysis drew attention to some of the characteristics of an outbreak of plague, there was no reason to reconsider the regulations in the intervals between the major epidemics. Only when they were put to the test could their effectiveness be assessed and, if found wanting, alternative strategies be devised. Thus, during the mid-1660s the government first ordered the implementation of the measures previously employed and then was forced to reappraise them, as the epidemic produced both large numbers of deaths and economic dislocation, affecting its own revenues and ability to carry on the war with the Dutch.

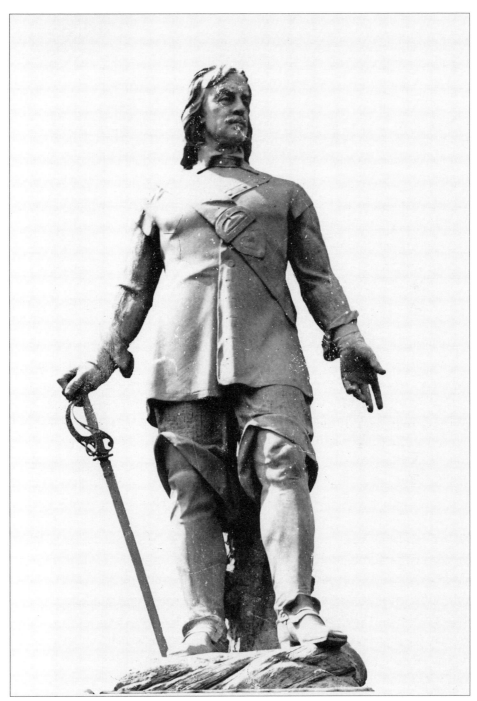

Quarantine regulations were put in place by the Protectorate government in 1655. Matthew Noble's model for his statue of Oliver Cromwell stood in Parliament Square for a short time in 1871. (© Crown copyright, NMR)

As the threat of plague grew in the early 1660s, the Privy Council began to consider what steps should be taken to prevent it spreading to Britain. The quarantining of shipping was the obvious policy, a method employed by Charles I's government thirty years earlier, and again by the Protectorate in the 1650s. The instructions issued by the Council of State in 1655 had been that no one from vessels arriving at English ports should be allowed to land until it had been established where they were from, and if from the Netherlands then they should be kept in quarantine for twenty days. Even when they had served the period of quarantine without showing any symptoms of the disease, they were permitted to come ashore only in clothes brought from shore, and no goods were to be landed.[1] When in October 1663 the Privy Council responded to the threat posed by plague at Amsterdam and Hamburg and consulted the Lord Mayor, he recommended the adoption of similar procedures, following not only the precedents of the 1630s and 1650s but also 'the example of other Countries'. Thomas Chiffinch, Groom of the Chamber to Charles II, also made a submission along those lines, arguing that such a policy was generally employed, except by the Turks, who took no preventive measures because of their fatalism. He made the case for the issue of health certificates for anyone who was to land and the isolation of those who were sick, at first on board and then by being kept apart on shore.[2]

In November a rigorous system of regulation was introduced to protect London, with two of the Navy's ships patrolling the Thames estuary to intercept all incoming vessels and ascertain where they were from. The masters of those from Amsterdam, Hamburg or any port known to be infected were to be given the choice of turning back to sea or performing quarantine for thirty days at Hole Haven on Canvey Island, where a lazaretto was to be established. When a vessel was serving its period of quarantine, a Navy ketch would patrol the entrance to the haven. Those ships which had come from places free from the plague were given certificates of health by the captains of the patrolling ships, and the commanders of the fort at Tilbury and the blockhouse at Gravesend on the south side of the Thames, opposite Tilbury, were instructed not to allow any vessel to pass unless they had such a certificate. The system thus provided a double cordon, for should any vessel be missed by the patrols in the estuary, they would be halted at Tilbury or Gravesend. No exceptions were made for vessels from Holland, for the Council ruled that 'noe Passenger permitted to be wafted over into England in the Pacquet boat' from Scheveningen, or any Dutch port.[3]

The policy was employed flexibly and adapted to changing conditions. In January 1664 the restrictions on shipping from Hamburg were lifted when the

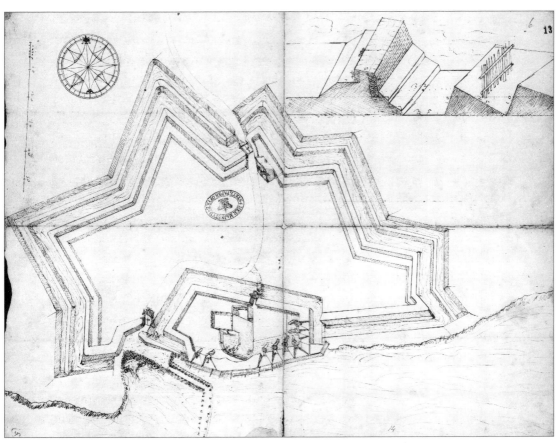

As part of the quarantine regulations, the garrison of Tilbury Fort checked shipping coming towards London. (Courtesy of the Public Record Office, London. SP 12/217/13)

Council was assured that the epidemic in the city had ended, although they were reimposed in July on the information that the plague was again prevalent there, before being revoked once more at the end of November. Similarly, the area of origin of those vessels required to serve quarantine was extended to encompass all ports in Holland and Zeeland, and later those in Friesland as well, on the realisation that Amsterdam had regular commerce with such ports, and that the epidemic in the Netherlands was worsening. With the spread of the plague there and the approach of the warmer weather 'which renders the contagion more dangerous', in May the quarantine period was lengthened to forty days. The prohibition on the landing of people or goods from vessels coming from Dutch ports was also applied to other ports in England and Wales, initially at Great

Yarmouth, where the corporation was recommended to adopt 'the Method observed here in the River of Thames', and then by orders addressed to twenty-eight other ports around the coast. The policy was successful enough to elicit a complaint from the Dutch ambassador that it was impeding the free passage of people and goods, and so damaging the trade of both countries. The Privy Council was sympathetic, but pointed out that its chief concern was the protection of the population 'which cannot be done without such restraints' and that Britain had been the last of the United Provinces' neighbours to impose restrictions. It then proceeded to extend them, by prohibiting the admission of all vessels coming from ports in Holland and Zeeland between the end of August and December.[4]

Applications for exemptions from the strict enforcement of the quarantine procedure also suggest that it had been largely effective. Evasion had been a problem in 1655, when it had been objected that the effect had been to increase avoidance of customs dues. Some flouting of the regulations occurred again during 1664, with sailors from vessels from Holland going ashore without serving a period of quarantine. The Council's reaction was to order the Justices of the Peace to secure those who were found to have ignored the regulations and to shut up for forty days houses where they or their goods had been lodged.[5] On the other hand, the impounding at Hole Haven of such varied cargoes as sixteen horses from Friesland for the royal service, Rhenish wines, barrels of cod and peas, glazed tiles for the king's palace at Greenwich, cordage and barrel staves, indicates that vessels which were intercepted were treated strictly. Some exemptions were allowed, as in the case of the cod and peas, which were perishable, and essential naval stores in the Thames and at Yarmouth. Yet in other cases the Council allowed no more than a moderation of the regulations, by permitting the goods or passengers to be landed but stipulating that the outstanding period of isolation should be served in full ashore. A heavily pregnant woman who had come from Hamburg aboard a ship that was then kept for three weeks near Rochester was permitted to land, but only if no one on board was sick, and with only one maid. They were required to serve another two weeks ashore without any contact, except in a case of 'absolute necessity'.[6]

The quarantine system in the Thames estuary was maintained throughout 1664 and may be judged to have been successful, as it had been in 1655, with only a very few cases of plague recorded in London in each of those years. It may have been less effective at Yarmouth, if the beginning of the epidemic there during the autumn of 1664 was indeed caused by infection brought from Rotterdam. Yet the concern of the Privy Council, which had been evident from late in 1663, appears to have lessened in the early months of 1665. This was not because of dissatisfaction with the policy or doubts regarding its effectiveness. Indeed, the added advantages of the system were recognised: ensuring the payment of customs dues; facilitating the regulation of imports; assisting marketing through the information that it provided of what merchandise was in port; and identifying which travellers were merchants. But the Council's attention became focused rather on the growing tension with the United Provinces, the seizure of merchantmen and the slide towards war, which was declared in March, than on health precautions. The need for quarantine was reduced, at least in respect of commerce with the Netherlands, by the deterioration of relations and accompanying breakdown in trade, and more widely by the Privy Council's order for ships engaged in overseas trade to be kept in port over the winter. The order was lifted at the end of November, except for the vessels of Dutch owners, but reimposed in mid-December. Its purpose presumably was to make their crews available for impressment into the Navy in the spring. Furthermore, the States General instructed Dutch ships not to enter English ports, to avoid seizure. Such a decrease in overseas trade, especially with the Netherlands, may have produced a decline in vigilance in the spring of 1665 that allowed a vessel carrying the infection to enter the Thames. After the plague had appeared in London, the Council's policy necessarily shifted from the exclusion of the disease to its containment.[7]

When plague was identified in St Giles-in-the-Fields, the Privy Council ordered the justices to take what measures they thought necessary to contain the disease, specifying only the shutting up of houses. In May a committee of the Council was formed to deal with the emerging problem. Its earliest orders were concerned with those two common targets of seventeenth-century governments, alehouses – the numbers of which were to be reduced – and inmates, or lodgers, who were regarded as a cause of overcrowding and the unhealthy conditions that it produced. Laws against inmates were in place, and they were to be enforced.[8] The committee also issued a series of instructions to the justices of Westminster and Middlesex, dealing with general matters regarding cleanliness and specific ones making provision for plague victims. Laystalls near to public thoroughfares were to be to be removed, ditches were to be cleansed, every householder was to be instructed to keep the street in front of his house clean 'all the weeke long', and rubbish was to be taken away daily. Dogs, cats, hogs, tame pigeons and rabbits were prohibited and dogs were to be disposed of by a dog-killer appointed for the

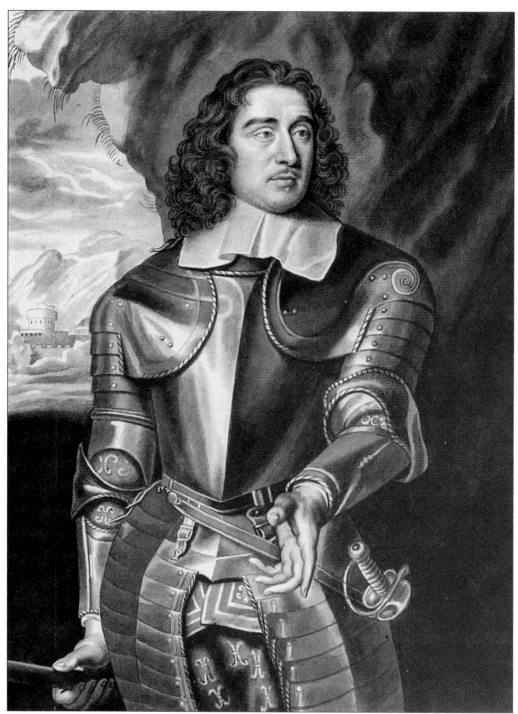

George Monck, Duke of Albemarle, remained at Westminster during the Great Plague.
(© Ashmolean Museum, University of Oxford)

purpose. Pigs found in public places were to be impounded. Regulation also extended to the sale of produce, with an order that no 'stinking fish or unwholesome flesh musty corne or other corrupt fruites' should be sold and brewers' premises and tippling houses should be inspected for 'musty and unwholesome casks'. Bread was regarded as posing a risk and so an order was issued that it should not be taken from bakehouses while it was still hot. The danger of the disease being spread in fabrics prompted a ban on street-sellers hawking old clothes and shopkeepers displaying them for sale.[9]

In addition to concern with environmental conditions, the committee also considered the provision for plague victims and those suspected of carrying the disease. The parish of St Margaret, Westminster, already had a pest-house, but it was occupied by 'sundry persons'. They were to be removed and the justices were instructed to see that the building was fitted up for its proper purpose, and they were also to supervise the erection of a new pest-house between Tyburn and Tottenham Court. The closing of houses occupied by plague suspects and those who may have been in contact with the disease was a further conventional element in the policy being promoted by the committee. Churchwardens were to ensure that those who were incarcerated should not converse with anyone outside the house, and those who visited the sick, such as physicians and searchers, were not only forbidden to go to public gatherings, but were required to carry a white wand, roughly 4 ft long, so that others could avoid them. Public funerals were prohibited.[10] Similar steps were taken by the corporation, which reprinted the plague *Orders* issued in earlier epidemics, most recently in 1646. The measures which the aldermen were enjoined to see observed included ensuring that the streets were kept clean, the need to report deaths from plague in order to avoid falsification of the returns, and the prevention of gatherings at burials.[11] Clarendon was particularly exasperated by attendance at funerals, in defiance of orders to the contrary that should have been read in every church, fearing that 'goinge to publique buryalls must infecte the whole kingdome'.[12] Other functions likely to attract crowds were also undesirable, especially fairs, which drew large numbers and from a wide area. In June the St James's Day fair at Bristol and Stourbridge fair at Cambridge were prohibited, and in August fairs within a radius of fifty miles of the capital were banned and Londoners were forbidden to attend any fairs. Other fairs were prohibited as the epidemic spread.[13]

As the numbers of victims in London grew and towns elsewhere reported the appearance of plague, there was little the government could do other than monitor its progress and urge the enforcement of the regulations. These were put in place, but their effectiveness relied on the determination and ability of the county justices and borough magistrates. Even when those authorities had specified the measures that should be taken, their implementation was in the hands of the officers who were to enforce them. Thus, the efficacy of the policy on plague was dependent on the conscientiousness, and indeed the courage, of individual churchwardens, constables and watchmen. Not only did they have to run the risk of contracting the disease, but also to suffer assaults by those who resented being delayed or prevented from carrying on with their normal routines. One man was charged with 'assaulting and striking' a parish constable who had questioned him, suspecting that he was bringing goods into the parish from a house in St Giles-in-the-Fields without a health certificate.[14]

The task of such officers in implementing the measures adopted was not made easier when those ultimately responsible for their enforcement decamped. While some aldermen and councillors in stricken towns stayed on and attempted to maintain direction of the administration, others, such as those at Norwich and Great Yarmouth, left their officers to carry out instructions. The role of the justices formed a major element in the plague policies of the Stuart governments, but it was an insecure one. Sir Theodore de Mayerne had envisaged them taking control and exercising 'absolute power' when an epidemic struck. In practice, they often appear to have been more active in directing the setting up of quarantine arrangements when plague threatened than supervising the collection of rates when it had broken out.[15] Their absence from a stricken community not only left a void in the direction of measures to contain the disease but also provoked resentment. This surfaced in a number of places, and fuelled one of the government's major concerns during the epidemic, which was fear of disorder, probably whipped up by the nonconformists. In practice, the small number of officers appointed to enforce the orders were faced not with unrest borne of political or religious discontent, but behaviour resulting from the effects of the policies on plague. They could not hope to deal with a recalcitrant population unwilling, out of economic necessity, to observe restrictive regulations. Their efforts required cooperation and perhaps, too, perceptible evidence that the policies were effective. By the summer of 1665 it was all too obvious in London, and indeed elsewhere, that this was not the case.

The failure of the measures taken to contain the outbreak in the capital led to a reconsideration of their value. In particular, the policy of isolating suspects in their houses was called into question. Its social unfairness was one aspect that aroused hostility, with the few who gave the 'Cruel Direction' to shut up houses able to retire to their 'Country-Gardens', leaving 'many thousand poor Innocents' to be incarcerated, with only such allowance for subsistence as the parish could afford. Why could the procedure not be applied uniformly? Thus, if someone died who had attended a meeting of the parish vestry, then surely 'the doors should be shut upon the Assembly', or the others who had been there ought to be quarantined in their houses. This was presumably the logic behind an attempt to shut up the Lord Mayor's own house in St Helen's, Bishopsgate for which several men were bound over to appear at the sessions.[16]

Those who were likely to be condemned to a 'miserable, noisome, melancholy, close imprisonment' in their houses were motivated by the same sense of self-preservation as those who imposed the policy and then withdrew to safety. The author of *The Shutting up Infected Houses as it is practised in England Soberly Debated* pointed out that they, too, had recourse to flight, thereby 'scattering the infection along the streets' as they went and leaving their families to the support of the parish. Shutting up a house had to be done quickly once the plague had been identified, if the action was to be effective. Allowing the occupants to continue to circulate and buy provisions risked spreading the disease. Thus, those who were confined to their houses were often unprepared and reliant on what could be supplied to them. This was one of the reasons for a reluctance to admit to a suspicious illness, and so it often happened that a house was not closed until an occupant had died, probably after the infection had been spread. Such lack of confidence in the arrangements for feeding and nursing the sick made enforcement of the policy difficult. But this could be overcome, it was argued in one report, by the provision of medical assistance and payments to compensate those who were incarcerated for the loss of their earnings. These could be drawn from a fund administered by commissioners approved by the king.[17]

Even if such practicalities could be managed efficiently, the basis of the practice was still open to question, especially the confinement of those who were healthy with those who were sick. With such a contagious disease, to sequester the occupants in this way was to put their lives at risk and almost inevitably to increase the death toll. This was partly because to seal up a house for the statutory forty days created the conditions which were thought to facilitate the spread of plague. The 'unquenchable stench, and fest' produced would invariably be dispersed, from the windows, or when the doors were unsealed to admit the searchers and bearers. This exposed a major contradiction in the measures taken against the disease, enjoining cleanliness wherever possible and yet creating an insanitary environment by compelling people to remain together in a confined space. The conditions thought to favour plague were to be found in the very houses that were sealed in order to prevent its transmission, so that the 'Infection may have killed its thousands, but shutting up hath killed its ten thousands.'[18]

Not only were the environmental conditions conducive to the spread of plague but so, too, were the psychological ones. Nathaniel Hodges wrote that 'the consternation of those who were separated from all society, unless with the infected, was inexpressible' and this, he believed, 'made them but an easier prey to the devouring enemy'. Their gloom could not but be intensified when their incarceration was prolonged if, for example, a new case was suspected in a house just before the period of quarantine was due to end, requiring all the occupants to endure a further term. Hodges poured out his righteous indignation against the practice, which he regarded as 'abhorrent to religion and humanity'. William Boghurst drew similar conclusions, noting that being shut up 'bred a sad apprehension and consternation' on those who were confined, and that 'one friend growing melancholy for another' in those circumstances was a reason for the plague spreading through a family.[19]

The views of senior churchmen were expressed in the 'Exhortation Fit for the Time' that accompanied the *Form of Common Prayer* for the fast days. It enjoined sensible behaviour and condemned those who acted in a careless and fatalistic way by going 'desperately and disorderly into all places, and amongst all persons, and pretend our faith and Trust in Gods providence', for this smacked of Satan tempting Christ to throw himself from the temple. Those who had the disease should act charitably towards their fellow citizens and not disobey authority by mixing with others, 'whereby the mortality daily so increaseth'. Such behaviour was all the more reprehensible because those who were infected were 'the meanest among the people' and yet 'think scorn to keep their houses' and break out, regardless of the consequences. While this was condemned as being a wilful defiance of authority, the authors of the 'Exhortation' also recognised that it was often necessary, for those who were incarcerated could be deprived of an adequate supply of provisions. Their conclusion was that there had to be care to keep those who were ill separate from those who were well, but that close confinement was self-defeating, for those within the houses that were shut up 'will break forth for the succour of their lives', and no authority or orders could restrain them. The solution was for the wealthy to play their part in the process by making generous contributions towards maintaining the poor who were confined.[20]

Dissatisfaction with the policy appears to have been widespread, but what were the alternatives to the isolation of households, which was, after all, one of the

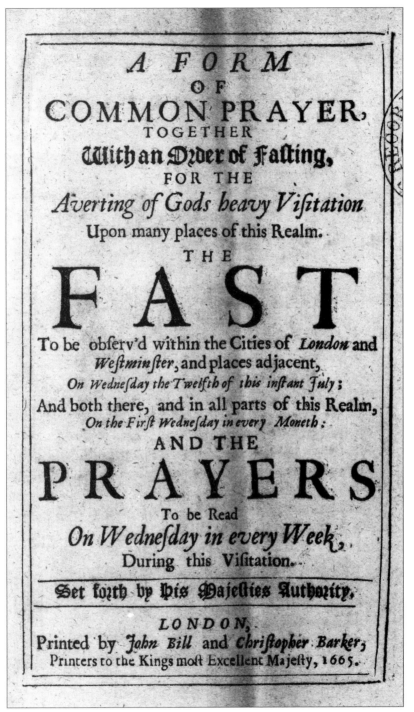

A form of Common Prayer with an Order of Fasting were issued for use during the plague.
(Courtesy of the Public Record Office, London. SP 29/126/65)

fundamental components of the government's strategy? Sir William Petty's imaginative solution was a large-scale evacuation of London's population to the surrounding area where, he calculated, there were as many houses as in the city.[21] Within a thirty-five mile radius of the capital 'large wide roomey' detached houses could be prepared, each having a water supply and a garden, and the inhabitants, who would be given seven days' notice of moving, could be transported to them in 'Convenient wagons or coaches'. According to his calculations this would be cost-effective; the expense of moving and lodging the evacuees would be £50,000, yet the value of each individual killed in the epidemic he calculated to be £7, producing a total of £840,000 if, as he anticipated, the next great plague of London claimed 120,000 victims. Although his solution may have seemed an impractical one, similar schemes of mass evacuation had been implemented by some Italian cities in the 1570s, albeit using less salubrious accommodation than that envisaged by Petty. The government of Venice had moved those citizens most at risk to 1,200 huts on an island in the lagoon, and some of the Milanese poor were transferred to huts made of wood or straw.[22] Petty evidently was dissatisfied with the effectiveness of the policy of shutting up some suspected of having plague in their houses and moving others to pest-houses close to the city, and was also aware that the remedies of killing dogs, lighting fires in the streets and taking medicines were not 'considered sure'. He argued against the complacent, and chilling, opinion that the death toll in an epidemic was 'but a seasonable discharge of its Pestilent humour'. If the plague distinguished between those who supported and those who opposed peace and obedience, or between the bees and the drones, then 'the Fact would determine the Question', but if it destroyed without distinction, then the country lost the productive contribution of the victims.

Such doubts about the existing policies were not so strongly expressed by the Earl of Craven when, in February 1666, he reported to the Privy Council the measures that had been taken since the previous spring, and the difficulties encountered.[23] He was well placed to make an assessment of the effectiveness of the policy set out by the Council during the previous spring and summer, having supervised its implementation, under the authority of the Duke of Albemarle. Writing four days after attending a meeting of the Middlesex justices, Craven first drew attention to the problems of disposing of the dead. The opening of new burial grounds had been limited by the Bishop of London's unwillingness to consecrate them unless the title to the site had been obtained. Practical problems had also arisen with interments in churchyards, for the price and scarcity of lime had restricted its use. Nevertheless, fresh earth and lime had been spread in many

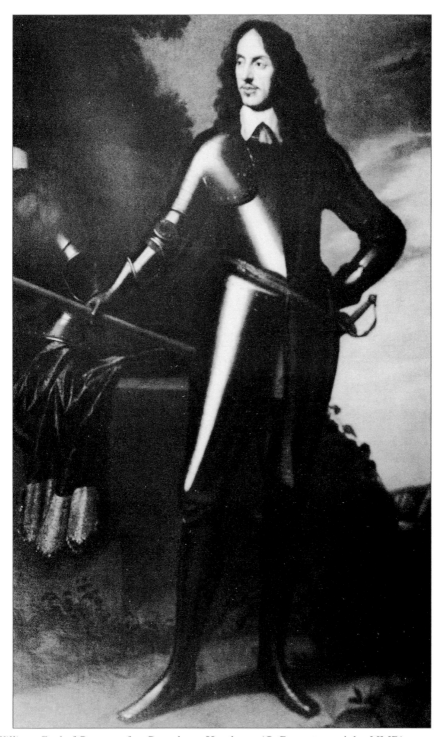

William, Earl of Craven, after Gerard van Honthurst. (© Crown copyright, NMR)

of them, and bodies buried at such a depth 'that we hope no inconvenience can from thence arise', especially as the graves were not to be reopened. Craven then considered the implementation of the orders concerning cleanliness. Those instructions regarding the removal of garbage from the streets had been observed, with the carts passing along every morning, also giving householders the chance to dispose of their domestic rubbish. On the other hand, he had to admit to 'many difficulties' in trying to get laystalls moved away from thoroughfares. Evidently this had not been too successful, but he was hopeful that the justices would be able to clear those which remained.

The success of the policies concerning beggars and inmates had also been mixed. While beggars had been removed and punished, the justices' instructions to eject inmates could not be implemented quite so easily, for although beggars

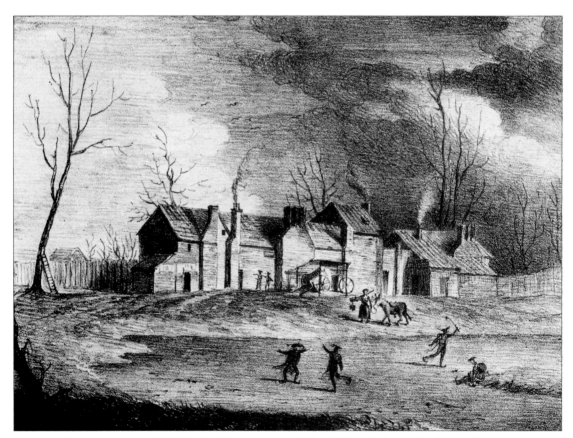

The pest-house at Tothill Fields, Westminster, c. 1840. (© The Wellcome Institute Library, London)

could be dealt with 'according to law', many inmates held 'particular leases and contracts' granted by the householders with whom they were lodged. As with laystalls, tenurial rights circumscribed the ability of the justices to implement the Privy Council's orders. They were, in any case, aware of the consequences of enforcing a policy which would have the effect of making 'poor necessitous persons' dependent on the relief that could be dispensed by the parishes, at a time when they were least able to provide it. Despite such reservations, at their meeting in February the justices had reissued the regulations directed at the removal of inmates with an order that stipulated that houses which had been divided should be reconverted into single dwellings and inmates expelled from all buildings, with the aim that only one family should live in each house.[24] In the same month, the Privy Council directed the corporation to clear inmates from houses, 'as a thing of very great Moment'. Just three months later the MP William Prynne pointed out that the implementation of the policy had caused discontent, with complaints that its effects would be worse than those of the plague. He also challenged the wisdom of the measure, pointing out that the expulsion of inmates would remove those who were too poor to rent an entire house, or who required only small and temporary lodgings, thereby depriving employers of their labour and reducing landlords' rental incomes.[25]

In his report Craven drew particular attention to the role of the pest-houses, which he regarded as 'the most probable means of hindering the spreading of the contagion', and the inadequate accommodation provided in them. He had taken the initiative during the epidemic to help to remedy the shortage of space in the pest-houses, by acquiring first a lease and later the freehold of a plot of ground in St James's, Westminster. There he erected a pest-house, described in 1739 as 'thirty-six small Houses, for the Reception of poor and miserable Objects . . . afflicted with a direful Pestilence, Anno 1665'.[26] Even with this addition, there were few places in the pest-houses, compared to the numbers of victims. That in Soho could hold just ninety people and the one in St Giles-in-the-Fields had space for only sixty, in a parish with 'multitudes of poor'. Indeed, the five pest-houses around London in 1665 could hold fewer than 600 people. Given the burden of taxes and parish rates, the financial problems of the 'middling people' because of the plague, and the absence of the wealthy, simply maintaining the existing pest-houses was likely to be a problem, let alone further resources being required for their enlargement. This was a matter which Craven referred to the Council, asking for aid, having described the role of the pest-houses during the epidemic as receiving those infected 'who were removable'. When appointed to

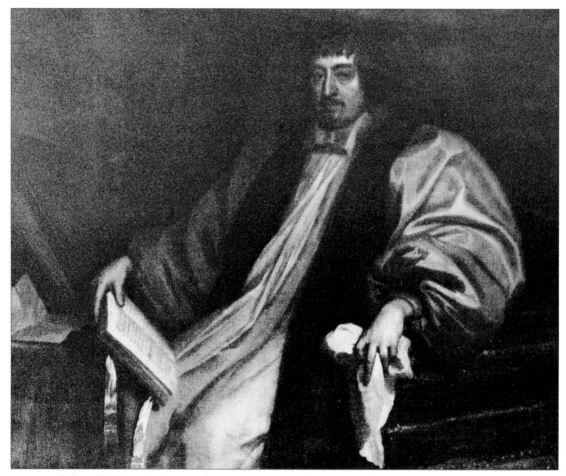

Gilbert Sheldon, Archbishop of Canterbury 1663–77, after Sir Peter Lely. (© Crown copyright, NMR)

the Privy Council's committee for the plague in May, Craven repeated his belief that plague was spread not by the air, but by the failure 'in the beginning' to remove from their houses those suspected of having the disease. From his experience of the plague in London, he concluded that the key to limiting an outbreak was to have adequate and well-provided pest-houses.[27]

While Craven's analysis of the role of pest-houses was sensible his summary of the way in which the policy of household isolation was carried out was highly questionable, for he reported that there had been 'no complaints brought to the justices of any neglect therein' and that they believed that 'due execution hath been generally made of this order, having themselves made a particular observation in several places'. This contradicts both the general impression, expressed by Pepys and Vincent among others, that the system had not only been challenged but had actually broken down, and also the evidence of cases that had come to the justices' attention. These included an incident in which a weaver had torn the lock off the door of a house in St Stephen, Coleman Street where a friend was quarantined; another that involved a woman of St Giles-in-the-Fields for 'opening and entring a house infected'; and examples of goods being moved from houses containing plague victims. At the very beginning of the epidemic, the Council had been made aware of the opening of a building in St Giles-in-the-Fields 'in a riotous manner' so that the occupants, who should have been held in quarantine, had been able to leave and mix with others. Despite Craven's account, the Privy Council could hardly have failed to be aware both of the shortcomings of the system and the opposition which it had aroused. Nevertheless, its directions to magistrates in the early months of 1666 showed no change in its policy, although they did stress the importance of the pest-houses.[28]

The Council's procedures regarding plague were codified in its Rules and Orders, issued in May and directed to all justices, mayors and bailiffs.[29] These contained many regulations already in force, such as those regarding certificates of health for visitors and goods, a ban on travelling vagabonds and beggars, and the prohibition of public gatherings, including funerals and wakes, in any place where plague was suspected. Fire was to be provided 'in movable Pans, or otherwise' where 'necessary publique Meetings' were held, for instance in churches. The need for cleanliness both in public places and houses was reiterated, and it was ordered that pigs, dogs, cats and tame pigeons were not to be permitted to wander around the streets or go from house to house, but there was no requirement that they should be killed. Previous regulations regarding burials of plague victims were extended with an order that prohibited them in churches and churchyards altogether, unless the churchyard was so large that a space could be set aside for such interments and was surrounded by a fence 10 ft high. Despite objections to the practice of expelling inmates, the Rules and Orders included a directive that the law against them should be enforced.

A significant modification in policy was made regarding isolation, supporting Craven's conclusions by giving prominence to the role of pest-houses. It was ordered that a pest-house, huts or sheds be provided in every town and that those who were sick should be removed there 'forthwith . . . for the preservation of the rest of the family'. A house from which the sick had been taken should then be closed and guarded for a forty-day period, with warders appointed to provide supplies for the occupants, as well as 'to keep them from conversing with the sound'. When the house was opened, strangers could not be lodged there for a further forty days, and no clothing or household goods removed within three months. By ordering the segregation of those who were ill, this measure did meet the objections of those who condemned the shutting up of the sick with the healthy. Of course, for the system to be effective the pest-houses had to be large enough to accommodate all plague victims, and in a major epidemic they were likely to be deluged. The policy also depended on adequate preparations and the prompt removal of those who showed the symptoms of the disease. If this were done, then such an eruption could be prevented, although recent experience showed that even cities which had large-scale quarantining facilities nevertheless suffered devastating outbreaks of plague, most recently Genoa in 1656–7 and Amsterdam in 1663–4.

A major stumbling block to the operation of the policy of isolation in the past had been the reluctance of those with plague symptoms to cooperate by volunteering themselves for internment. In order to meet the objections that those who were quarantined faced deprivation because of the inability of the authorities to maintain them, the Rules and Orders made provision for financial relief for those communities unable to support their sick. The justices were given authority to levy a rate on the nearby parishes without delay, to be confirmed at the next quarter sessions. Adequate support would not only reassure those who faced isolation, but also prevent the conditions which were perceived to be among the reasons for the spread of the plague, 'want and nastiness being great occasions of the Infection'. Here was a major reason for tying in the action against inmates to plague control, for they were regarded as being 'poore indigent and idle and loose persons' who placed such a strain on poor relief that 'the wealthy are not able to relieve the poore in times of health', and even less so during an epidemic. Without the burden which they imposed on the system, more resources could be directed to the poor who were sick.[30]

The justices' powers to set an emergency rate in such circumstances were not new, but were a restatement of a measure that had been given parliamentary sanction in an Act of 1604. That Act was designed to overcome the problem of providing charity for the poor plague victims, by giving the justices authority to levy rates within the affected community and, if the sums raised were insufficient, to extend the collection to the area within a radius of five miles. With that provision in place, those who were confined to their houses had no justification

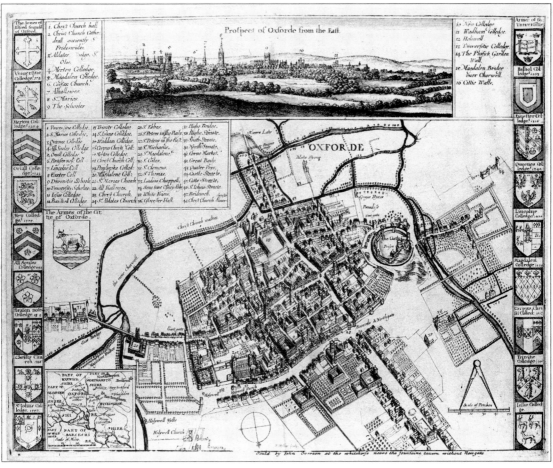

Because of the plague at Westminster, parliament assembled at Oxford in October 1665.
(© Ashmolean Museum, University of Oxford)

for attempting to go out, and so the watchmen were empowered 'with violence to inforce them to keep their houses' and given immunity 'if any hurt come by such inforcement'.[31]

The measures for financial assistance had not worked well under the strain of the epidemic in London in 1665, and the Oxford Parliament, meeting in October, set about dealing with the imperfections of the legislation. A committee of the House of Commons was appointed to consider the Act of 1604 and bring in a Bill that would remedy its shortcomings. The proposals were amended to some extent when they had been considered by the Lords, who queried clauses regarding pest-houses and churchyards and sought exemption for their own houses from shutting up. But on the day that the two Houses debated the Bill, the king prorogued parliament. Another Bill was introduced into the Commons a year later, reaching the committee stage by December and the Lords at the end of January 1667, but it, too, was lost. When it was debated by the two Houses the Commons pointed out that experience had shown that the Act of 1604 should be modified. Yet the Lords again attempted to exempt their houses from shutting up, a measure not included in that Act, and were opposed by the Commons, who argued that it would weaken the legislation rather than strengthen it. So many houses came within the peers' jurisdiction that to leave them unsealed when plague had been identified was to endanger the public. The Commons held it to be unreasonable that 'the People's Safety should depend upon their Lordships Pleasure to shut up themselves', making the obvious point that 'No dignity can exempt from Infection.' While they had no intention of reducing their lordships' privileges in this case, what was to be gained from insisting on such privileges when 'Death equals all'?[32]

The failure to get the Bill through all of the stages in October 1665, and the subsequent delays in recalling parliament – which was first scheduled to meet in the following February and then in April – may account for the timing of the Rules and Orders. Although the seasonal pattern of the disease was known, they were not issued until May, when the numbers of plague victims were already rising steeply in such towns as Colchester. Only if they had been produced and distributed during the winter months could they have been effective, giving the justices time to implement such arrangements as the provision of pest-houses before the upsurge of cases during the spring. Furthermore, the Privy Council had little choice but to adopt the financial provisions of the 1604 Act, if it were not to infringe parliament's rights. The legislation did not allow for the provision of an adequate fund from which those sequestered could be supplied with provisions, so that they were not dependent on such money as could be raised on the rates, nor did it grant enough powers to those collecting the rates. The problems therefore remained unresolved, especially of how to raise funds when the wealthy citizens had left; the rate-collectors feared for their lives in some streets where plague was present, and the economy was disrupted. Hence the reaction to the plague policies reported in London in 1665 were repeated in the worst-affected towns in the following year, and the spectre of widespread popular discontent remained.

In contrast to the Oxford Parliament's failure to tackle the issue of raising money for plague victims, it did respond to the problem created by the dispossessed clergy and the crown's need for funds to pursue the war with the Dutch. The ease with which nonconformist ministers who had been ejected from their livings since the Restoration had been able to move into the pulpits vacated by the clergy during the plague, especially in London, may have alarmed the senior churchmen. Their concern coincided with the government's fear of sedition, the danger of which had been increased by the withdrawal from the towns of many of the wealthier citizens and magistrates. Parliament, however, reacted not by strengthening the powers of the crown, but with a further measure designed to curb the influence of the nonconformists. The Five Mile Act required the ejected ministers to take an oath not to take up arms against the king or to attempt to try to alter the government of Church or state. Those who refused were forbidden to live within five miles of a corporate town or their former parishes, or to teach as a schoolmaster. The connection between the concern about sedition and the legislation was the assumption that the nonconformist preachers had the potential to foment discontent or even disorder, and that this was likely to occur, and to be most dangerous, in towns. A greater priority for the Oxford Parliament was to meet the government's needs for money to finance the war with the Dutch, to supplement existing revenues. It swiftly approved the levying of a further £1.25 million, to be raised by monthly assessments.[33] Yet collection of the new tax and the receipt of income from the regular revenues were both circumscribed by the economic dislocation caused by the plague. According to Clarendon, 'Monies could neither be collected nor borrowed where the plague had prevailed, which was over all the city and over a great part of the country; the collectors durst not go to require it or receive it.'[34]

Reluctance on the part of tax collectors to venture into areas where plague was present was both understandable and difficult to overcome. Furthermore, interruptions to inland and overseas trade, the quarantining of goods, cancellation of fairs, closure of workshops, the absence of groups of prosperous consumers, fear of plague and the high death toll, all contributed to the economic disruption. Health certificates were designed to prevent the breakdown of trade, by providing an assurance that goods had been brought from a place that was free of plague. Yet from the summer of 1665 and throughout 1666 the disease was so widespread across southern and much of eastern England that the system could not prevent a reduction in internal trade, and indeed of normal travel. Inns were best avoided, even in places which apparently were free from plague, making long-distance journeys difficult. Carriers stopped serving towns where the disease was present, perhaps for their own safety, but also because of the regulations imposed by the communities which they served, involving at least a period of quarantine and possibly the risk of confiscation. Farmers faced a similar difficulty in reaching their markets because of the health cordons around infected towns, and a longer-term one with the reduction in the number of urban consumers as a result of the high mortality.

The health regulations were bound to disrupt normal business. The Scottish Privy Council introduced strict measures, prohibiting traffic with Holland in 1664 and in July 1665 banning all trade with London and other infected places in England, both by sea and overland, subsequently extending the order until June 1666. The island of Inchkeith served as a quarantine station, with the period of isolation set at forty days, and masters who refused to take their vessels there were to be hanged and their cargoes burnt.[35]

The ports on the east coast of England also felt at risk and imposed controls on shipping coming from London and other infected ports, as well as from the United Provinces. While this kept some of them free from the disease, such as Whitby, Hull and Lowestoft, trade through them with their hinterlands was disrupted. With overland trade also subjected to restrictions, many places could not obtain those goods which they usually received from London. The most humble items were in short supply, such as the wax candles for services in Gloucester cathedral, for when the existing stock ran out they could not be brought from the capital 'by reason of that calamitie which of late hath hindered commerce with that place'. Postal services, too, were affected, as carriers ceased to travel. In the issue of its *Philosophical Transactions* dated 3 July 1665, the Royal Society anticipated that the printing of the journal would be suspended, because the epidemic 'may unhappily cause an interruption aswel of Correspondences, as of Publick Meetings'. Edward Wood sent two letters from Laleham to London in the second week of July 1665, but both were returned undelivered because the carrier had stopped operating his regular boat service along the Thames. The government itself found it difficult to overcome the problem of delays in the postal service. As late as mid-October mail from the north and west of England was still being sent to Oxford through London, producing delays.[36] The conduct of government business was made even more complex by the dispersal of its offices. The Exchequer and tally office were established at Nonsuch Palace near Ewell in mid-August 1665 and did not return until the following January, and the Navy Office was moved to Greenwich, although the Court of Admiralty was transferred to Winchester.[37]

The interruption of trade with London caused disruption over a large part of the country that was not confined to domestic production, for the capital handled roughly three-quarters of English overseas trade. Goods for export were shipped from its quays and imports brought in for distribution. Cloth formed a significant element, for not only did it account for about three-quarters of the capital's exports by value, but many of the finishing processes were carried out there. Conduct of business and the capital's foreign trade was hindered by the absence of many of the merchants. Most members of the East India Company's Committee left, and so could not meet 'to consider and directe affaires'.[38] Trade was also curtailed as foreign governments prohibited vessels coming from London. The ban introduced by the French authorities on all shipping going to the British Isles was especially damaging, for France accounted for one-sixth of London's trade.[39] Furthermore, in January 1666 France entered the war as allies of the Dutch. Both coastal and overseas trade became more hazardous as Dutch privateers made inroads into English merchant shipping, capturing perhaps as many as 500 vessels. The policy of the privateer captains was to seize all vessels trading to or from England, regardless of nationality. As the east coast was especially vulnerable to their depredations, the coal trade was seriously disrupted, but losses were not confined to vessels in the North Sea, for by June 1666 Bristol's merchants had lost 'the greatest part' of their ships.[40] Thus, the producing areas were cut off from their markets so long as the plague continued in London, and even when it had subsided there, cloth brought from those towns in East Anglia where the disease was still prevalent was held in quarantine for forty days before it could be taken into the city. As trade declined, foreign merchants saw no reason to remain. At the beginning of August 1665 the Dutch ambassador reported to the States General that many Dutch citizens were applying to leave London, as no trade was left there.[41]

Further dislocation was caused by the absence from London of the court and of the university from Cambridge. The court was a large and prosperous centre of consumption, and was arguably the single richest market in the country. Those traders and merchants who supplied it with both routine provisions and luxury goods were separated from their clients for the second half of 1665, and were unable to simply send their wares to Oxford because of the regulations imposed there. Nor could they find alternative customers among the gentry, the lawyers or the City's affluent élite, for many of them had left. They may, in any case, have had difficulty in obtaining supplies, for not enough produce reached the markets to allow buyers to be selective. The absence of the court and other wealthy

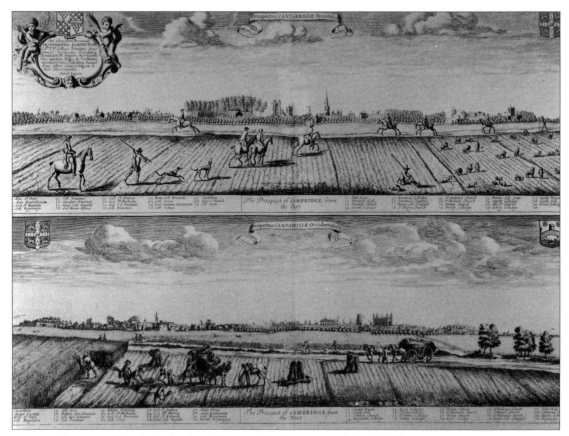

Prospects of Cambridge by David Loggan. (© Crown copyright, NMR)

elements brought unemployment and increased the pressure on the system of poor relief, especially in Westminster and the West End. Edmund Berry Godfrey complained that some of the nobility forgot their debts as well as their charity.[42] A similar situation obtained in Cambridge, where the absence of many members of the university and the siege mentality of those who remained had a damaging effect on the town's economy, producing a rapid increase in the numbers of the poor, 'in whome only we are rich'.[43] The pattern was repeated on a smaller scale in other towns, where the fear of plague led to the withdrawal of wealthy consumers.

As trade was disrupted, markets contracted and the plague threatened, workshops were closed because of the danger, the absence of the proprietors and the difficulties in moving the finished goods. Such closures were carried out swiftly, almost literally overnight. When plague was identified among the inhabitants of the houses in Old Gravel Lane off Houndsditch, Edward Wood wrote to John Pack early in August and recommended him to close their hemp-spinning workshop there and discharge the workmen. Some weeks later he discovered that Pack was still taking sugar into their warehouse in Thames Street, and so directed him 'to keepe the shopp dores shutt . . . 'tis better to loose the warehouse rent than to hazard your health'.[44] During an epidemic the risk to life took precedence over the drive for profit. As a result, the towns that were affected experienced very swift increases in the numbers unemployed, as economic activity was severely reduced. In July 1666 Thomas Corie thought that within three weeks at least 3,000 people in Norwich would be out of work and at Cambridge the poor were estimated to number more than 4,000 – half the population – while by the beginning of 1667 roughly one-third of the inhabitants of Salisbury were receiving relief.[45]

The disruption was also reflected in sharp falls in production and trade. Fines collected by the officers of the Dutch Bay Hall for substandard workmanship provide an indication of the output of bays at Colchester. The annual average for 1661–5 was £89, but in 1666 only £31 was collected and in 1667 £61, suggesting that cloth production in the town fell by about a half during the epidemic. Ipswich's trade showed a similar decline. Tolls taken at the quay on incoming coal, corn and salt averaged £12 per annum between 1659 and 1664, but just £5 was collected in 1665 and £6 in 1666.[46] Even places that escaped the plague were caught up in the recession, especially those in the hinterlands of towns that were infected. In Sudbury, sixteen miles from Colchester and twenty-two from Ipswich, the large numbers of poor there were blamed on 'a great decay of Trade by reason of the Sickness & Plague which is in most of the adjacent Townes'.[47]

The economic impact of the plague was especially apparent in London. Before the end of July Pepys noticed that the streets were 'mighty thin of people' and when he travelled across the City from Whitehall to Seething Lane on one occasion he passed just two coaches and two carts along the way. In August he estimated that at least two-thirds of the shops in his neighbourhood were shut. By late September only 'poor wretches' were to be seen in the streets; he would encounter fewer than twenty people while walking the length of Lombard Street, and grass was growing in Whitehall Court. The City had become 'like a place distressed – and forsaken'. Pepys noted, too, that there were 'no boats upon the River' and when he met Sir George Carteret in November he watched with interest Sir George's reaction when he saw 'the river so empty of boats'. The

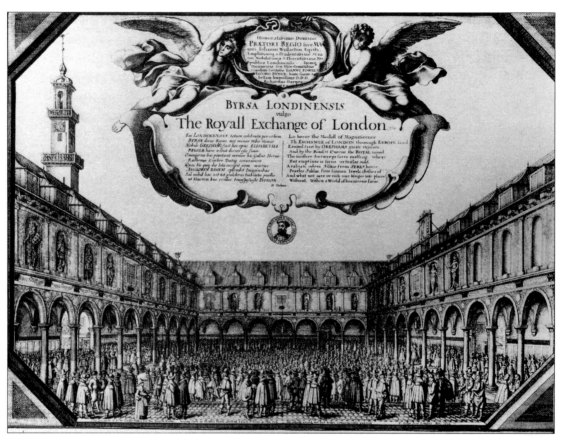

Wenceslaus Hollar's view of the Royal Exchange, 1644. (© Crown copyright, NMR)

Royal Exchange was at the heart of the mercantile community in London, the place where much of its business was transacted. Hollar's view of 1644 shows the courtyard thronged with several hundred people, an accurate reflection of the numbers who regularly appeared there. Yet as the plague worsened the numbers fell away sharply. Before the end of July they were 'very thin' and when Pepys was there at the end of August he thought that there were no more than fifty people in all. Thus, he was surprised a few weeks later to find as many as 200, but he noted another factor, which was that the crowd did not include 'a man or merchant of any fashion, but plain men all', and again in October it was being frequented by 'but mean people'.[48]

The absence of the wealthier merchants and goldsmiths was significant so far as the government was concerned, because it hampered its attempts to raise money to finance the war with the Dutch. Few men who were left had the resources to provide loans or advance sums in anticipation of tax revenues.[49] Pepys discussed the problem with the wealthy goldsmith Sir Robert Viner, and they came to the depressing conclusion that there was 'no money got by trade' and that those in the City who had money could not 'be come at'. Viner protested his own shortage of funds and told Pepys that the yield from the hearth tax in London 'comes almost to nothing'.[50] This was bad news for the City corporation, which was assigned the receipts from both collections in 1665 and that at Lady Day 1666 as repayment of loans to the crown of £200,000. As London provided roughly 18 per cent of the yield from the tax, the difficulties there were not in

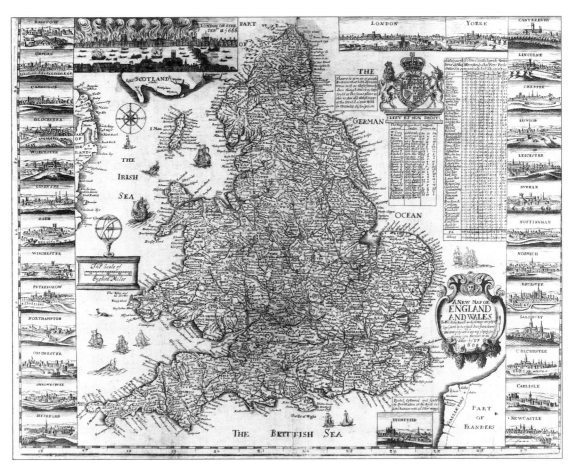

Robert Walton's map of England and Wales, 1668, with an inset depicting the Great Fire of London. (© Ashmolean Museum, University of Oxford)

themselves catastrophic, but as the plague spread so the problems of collecting the tax increased. By the end of 1666 approximately £100,000 had been received for the three collections, representing less than 60 per cent of the anticipated yield.[51]

The impact of the plague and the war on customs and excise revenues was equally severe. London accounted for 65–75 per cent of customs revenues and 30–40 per cent of those from the excise. The sharp fall-off in trade from the Thames was therefore bound to reduce the receipts from the customs, as were the problems faced by the other ports, both from the decline in traffic with the capital and the activities of the privateers. Indeed, the estimated shortfall was admitted by a government auditor to be more than £320,000, while the farmers responsible for collection claimed that the figure was nearer £400,000. Their estimates indicate that the loss was not far short of the anticipated yield for one year. The deficit for the excise was not as heavy, but nevertheless the figure of £88,000 that was allowed for the effect of the plague was one-third of the average annual yield in the preceding three years. The loss of potential revenue was divided between that which should have been drawn from London, which was valued at £70,000, and the provinces, with £18,000.

While the disruption of economic activity in places that suffered from the plague – coupled with the policy of suppressing alehouses – diminished the revenue from the excise, there were also some increases. The excise officers complained that between September 1666 and March 1667 receipts in Winchester were less than a quarter of their normal level, but because of the plague in London, Barnet and other towns in Hertfordshire attracted more business, producing an increase in excise receipts. But the plague also interfered with the collection of the two assessments: the Royal Aid, voted in 1664, and the Additional Aid, voted by the Oxford Parliament in October 1665. Revenue from the Additional Aid was particularly slow to come in, with only 59 per cent of the anticipated yield having been received by September 1667, its collection having been hampered by the effects of the plague. Given such losses, the net income of £281,000 from Dutch and French prizes was a comparatively small gain, although it had been hoped that such revenue would make an important contribution to the cost of the war.[52]

With such financial problems, the autumn of 1665 was a particularly difficult one for those struggling with the administration of the Navy. The Navy Board received no revenue for two months at the end of the campaigning season and the fleet was powerless to respond when the Dutch reappeared in the North Sea, so that they were able to cruise off the mouth of the Thames with impunity. Without money, the fleet could not be refitted and the crews retained, but nor could the seamen be paid when they were discharged. Most of them who were paid off were given tickets, which they had to redeem for cash at the best rate that they could find. Some were reduced to squatting outside the Navy Office, where Pepys was disconcerted by the 'lamentable moan of the poor seamen that lie starving in the streets for lack of money'.[53] Evelyn, too, was almost at his wit's end as he wrestled with the problem of trying to provide for nearly 10,000 wounded seamen and prisoners. When the two men and Evelyn's fellow Commissioners for the Sick and Wounded talked things over in September, they were pessimistic about the prospect of raising money during the epidemic. Things were so bad by the end of the month that Evelyn wrote that 'Our prisoners . . . beg us, as a mercy, to knock them on the head; for we have no bread to relieve the dying Creatures.'[54]

The plague impinged on the war effort not only through its contribution to the government's financial problems, but also by creating difficulties in provisioning and manning. Barrels were in short supply because of the number of coopers who had died in the plague or had moved away from London, leading to problems in victualling the fleet. The impact on manning came both from the number of deaths, reducing the potential numbers of sailors, and the risk of taking on board someone who was already infected. Isolation was virtually impossible to achieve on board a ship, and so there was a danger of plague spreading through an entire crew. Both merchant and naval captains were understandably cautious when manning their vessels, not accepting those who had been discharged as sick and wounded and had since recovered, nor those from infected areas. The rejection of men from places known to have plague victims was a serious restriction, given the prevalence of the disease in the riverside parishes of London in the second half of 1665 and in many towns on the lower Thames and the Medway in both 1665 and 1666. Manning remained a major problem throughout the war.[55]

The obstacles faced in the autumn of 1665 were tackled during the winter, as the plague in London diminished; the government could operate more normally, and the wealthy goldsmith bankers returned to the City. Loans were advanced to cover the immediate difficulties and the fleet was fitted out for sea in the spring of 1666. The summer campaigns saw a major engagement in early June, known as the Four Days Fight, and the St James's Day battle in July. Then in early September came the Great Fire of London, which destroyed 13,200 houses and 87 churches in the space of four days. In addition to the value of the buildings and goods that were destroyed, which were worth perhaps £8 million, trade through London was again disrupted and tax revenues were lost. During the following

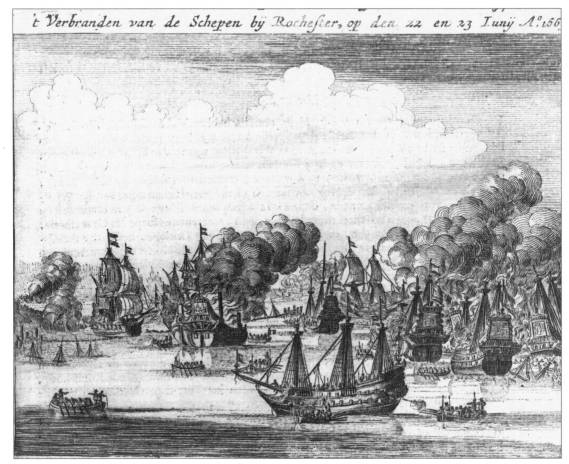

't Verbranden van de Schepen bÿ Rochester, op den 22 en 23 Iunÿ A°.156

The Dutch in the Medway, 1667, by Romeyne de Hooghe. (© National Maritime Museum, Greenwich, London)

winter the problems of finance and the provisioning of the Navy once more became acute. In the spring of 1667 the Navy Board realised that it could not send out the fleet, but would have to rely upon patrols by guard ships. The folly of the decision was brutally exposed by the Dutch, who raided the Medway, captured Sheerness, burnt three warships and towed away the flagship, *The Royal Charles*. The war came to an end in July with the Dutch fleet cruising off the mouth of the Thames, paralysing the capital's trade.[56]

Contemporaries tended to ascribe the depression of the years 1665–7 to the plague, the Great Fire and the war with the Dutch, without apportioning the effects of each. In fact, the coincidence of the plague and the fire with the war worsened, but did not cause, the problems of financing the campaigns. An indication of the extent to which the plague disrupted the economy, and hence contributed to the difficulties encountered in maintaining the war, may be judged from the loss of tax revenue attributed to the epidemic. The combined shortfall in the customs, excise and hearth tax was approximately £525,000, while the total cost of the war was ten times that sum, at approximately £5.25 million.[57] The outbreak also delayed the collection of other taxes and caused problems with provisioning and manning the fleet that could not be completely overcome.

The impact of the epidemic was, therefore, felt over much of the country and at many levels. Individuals suffered the loss of relatives and friends, household economies were disrupted by the enforcement of isolation and the loss of employment, many communities were affected by the dislocation of trade, and the government's efforts to maintain the fleet and wage war were impeded. The need for effective regulations was obvious, but the issue of the Rules and Orders in May 1666 came too late for those places which were already experiencing an upsurge of the disease. Preventive controls had also apparently been unsuccessful. Although effective in 1664, the regulation of incoming shipping failed to avert the outbreaks of the following years. Yet the experience did lead to an examination of the policies employed, which could be drawn upon in the future, as plague threatened once again.

CHAPTER 5

The Great Plague in Perspective

The City is outrageous, for you know, to merchants there is no plague so dreadful as a stoppage of their trade . . . I am in great apprehensions of our having the plague: an island, so many ports, no power absolute or active enough to establish the necessary precautions, and all are necessary! 'Tis terrible!

Horace Walpole to Sir Horace Mann, 31 July 1743

Despite the loss of life and the disruption of economic activity and the war effort, not everyone came to regard the Great Plague as an unmitigated disaster. Although some communities struggled to recover and later looked back on the plague years as having contributed to their problems, the fortunes of others revived fairly quickly. Individuals, too, found that the plague had created opportunities or perhaps a breathing-space, even though it had disrupted their lives. Indeed, some of those displaced by the epidemic were able to put their enforced break from their normal routines to good effect.

The plague years were an especially fruitful time for Isaac Newton, who later recalled that it had been a period when he was 'in the prime of my age for invention'. He graduated in the spring of 1665, left Cambridge for his family home at Woolsthorpe in June or July, returned to Trinity in the following March, but left again when the university was closed towards the end of June. He did not return until April 1667. According to his own chronology, during the plague years he conducted experiments refracting light through a triangular prism and evolved the theory of colours, invented the differential and integral calculus, and conceived the idea of universal gravitation, which he tested by calculating the motion of the moon around the earth. The story which Newton told William Stukeley in 1726, of how the fall of an apple, as he sat 'in contemplative mood', caused him to ponder why it should always descend perpendicularly, has traditionally been set in the orchard at Woolsthorpe, when he stayed there during the plague. It may be that, writing and reminiscing more than fifty years later, his recollections regarding the timing of these three major achievements were faulty, and the extent to which his stay in rural Lincolnshire because of the contagion in Cambridge contributed to his discoveries cannot be known, but the fact remains that a most important period in the history of European science coincided with the Great Plague.[1]

Less momentous, but not insignificant in terms of English literature, was the time which John Dryden spent at Charlton, his wife's family's estate in Wiltshire. This lasted for more than a year and proved to be a productive period during which he wrote the *Essay of Dramatick Poesie*, the play *Secret Love*, and the poem *Annus Mirabilis*, despite his protestation that in the country he was 'without the help of Books, or advice of Friends'. John Ogilby's retreat at Kingston-upon-Thames was less secluded, but he, too, used the time profitably, preparing a second volume of his paraphrases of Aesop's *Fables*.[2]

The return of those who, like Newton, Dryden and Ogilby, had temporarily moved away was an important stage in the recovery of communities that had been disrupted. With their reappearance, the previous patterns of economic and social behaviour could be resumed. Those places which had lost significant numbers of people during the epidemic, through death or departure, were able to recover by attracting immigrants and by natural replacement. The plague opened up opportunities for the survivors, by creating vacancies, drawing in those from outside who were able to move and take advantage of the openings. The process could begin quite soon after the end of the epidemic, when restrictions on movement were lifted and confidence returned. Demographic recovery took longer, as individuals picked up the threads of their lives. In its simplest form, the response was for those who had been widowed to remarry and start a new family, and for some couples who had lost children in the plague to have more. The age and health of the population, together with psychological factors, may have acted as constraints and could have been inimical to further births. Nevertheless, the expected pattern would be one of successive peaks of burials, marriages and baptisms.

The parish registers for Eyam show such a pattern. Following the high mortality in 1665 and 1666, far more marriages were celebrated there in the 1660s than during the preceding two decades. Although this trend had begun before the epidemic, the forty marriages recorded in 1667 and 1668 constituted the highest total for two successive years since the beginning of the registers in 1630. Similarly, the 187 baptisms in 1668–71 were the highest number in a four-year period since 1630. After 1671 the numbers declined, averaging 29.2 per annum for the remainder of the decade and 26.8 in the 1680s, compared with 28.8 in the 1640s and 30.6 in the 1650s. With burials during the 1670s and 1680s at roughly their pre-plague level, this pattern produced rising numbers, so that much of the loss during the epidemic had been replaced within a generation. This demographic revival seems to have been achieved without a high level of immigration. The increase came to an end around 1690, and the size of the population then stabilised, with little further growth in numbers in the 1690s. The gradual fall in the number of baptisms in the late seventeenth century could have been due to the 'missing' generation of children killed in the plague, although the births after the epidemic may have gone some way to replacing those lost. Social factors, not relating to plague, may also have had an effect. Nevertheless, both the speed of replacement of those who had died in the epidemic and the return to the demographic regime identifiable before 1665 are noteworthy, in a rural parish badly affected by the plague.[3]

At the other end of the scale, London experienced an even more remarkable recovery. The collectors of the hearth tax reported that the capital quickly filled up after the epidemic, and Nathaniel Hodges's impression was that the high mortality was 'after a few months . . . hardly discernable'.[4] These reactions are supported by the burial figures. The numbers in the *Bills* record a low of 12,697 in 1666 in the aftermath of the plague, which had carried off many of the most vulnerable, such as the elderly and the sick. The figure may also have been affected by the temporary displacement beyond the area of the *Bills* of some made homeless by the Great Fire. The number of burials in 1667 shows a marked rise, however, and was no lower than in 1663, and the mean annual return of burials in 1668–72 was 18,176, compared with 17,017 in 1660–4, a rise of almost 7 per cent. These were the years during which the houses destroyed in the Great Fire were replaced, with 8,000 erected by the end of 1672. The post-fire reconstruction brought in building workers and craftsmen from beyond London. Indeed, steps were taken to remove possible obstacles to their arrival by suspending the regulations restricting trading in the City to the citizens.[5] Even so, this influx does not explain immigration on the scale necessary to replace so quickly the numbers killed in the epidemic.

Urban areas tended to attract young single people, including many females who worked in domestic service, one of the groups which suffered high levels of mortality during the plague. It may be that much of the migration into London was accounted for by an acceleration of a continual process, with the replacement

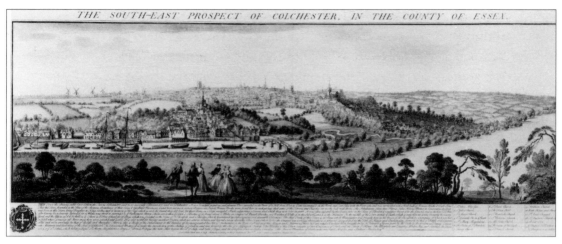

Colchester recovered its former prosperity after the epidemic of 1665–6. It is shown in this eighteenth-century view by Samuel and Nathaniel Buck. (© Crown copyright, NMR)

of domestic servants and apprentices who had died, and the re-establishment of households, as those who had temporarily moved away from the capital returned, bringing staff with them. Although most such immigrants would have been in the age group that experienced low mortality in normal conditions, and so would not be well represented in the burial record, those who remained, married and had children would have been recorded when their deaths, or those of their infants, were registered. Thus, the numbers of burials may provide a reliable guide to the size of the population and an indicator that, despite the scale of the mortality, the plague produced only a short-term loss of numbers in London. Such a swift recovery supports the conclusions of John Graunt, whose calculations, based on numbers of baptisms after the outbreak of 1625, led him to deduce that the population attained its former size by the second year after a major epidemic.[6]

Colchester's recovery also seems to have been a speedy one, for its population had risen to 9,500 by 1671 and may have reached 10,400 by 1674, not far short of the level before the plague in 1665–6. The evidence for cloth production indicates that the town's economy also revived with remarkable swiftness. Fines collected by the officers of the Dutch Bay Hall rose from £61 in 1667 to £101 in 1668 and averaged £124 per annum during the next five years, from 1669 until 1673, almost 40 per cent higher than the figure for the early 1660s. Such a revival could not have occurred without the replacement of much of the adult population lost in the epidemic, and suggests a high level of immigration into the town during

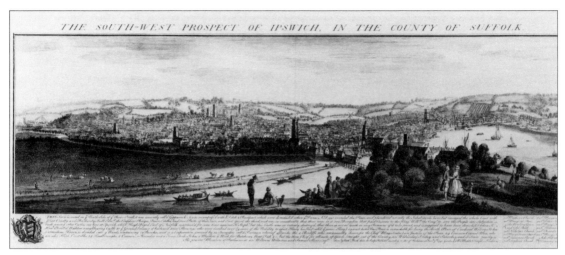

Ipswich is shown in Samuel and Nathaniel Buck's view of 1774. (© Crown copyright, NMR)

the late 1660s and early 1670s, as well as a maintenance of the skills required. The textile industry continued to be the principal source of employment during the late seventeenth century. Indeed, Colchester's economy saw little functional change during the period, with its coastal and overseas trade continuing to thrive. By the early eighteenth century the town was perceived to be populous and wealthy.[7]

Ipswich's population and economy took longer to recover, although its proportional loss in the plague had been less than at Colchester. Ipswich's demographic response to the losses in the epidemic was decidedly sluggish, with a surplus of just 322 baptisms over burials during the period 1667–73. The peak in baptisms after the epidemic was less prolonged than at Eyam and the number of burials stabilised at a much higher level than during the middle decades of the century. Furthermore, it seems that there was no considerable influx of immigrants, for an estimate of the population in 1674 produces a figure of 7,400, compared with 9,100 in 1664. This suggests a fall of 18 per cent over the ten years, or slightly more than the estimated loss in the plague. Shortly after the epidemic, in 1668 the corporation considered attempting to get Dutch linen makers and some manufacturers of white pottery ware to settle there, but nothing came of the proposal. During the second half of the seventeenth century the town's economy went through a period of adaptation, with its vessels increasingly engaged in coastal rather than overseas trade. Employment in shipping had been the largest occupational category before the Restoration, but was in relative decline thereafter, even though the tonnage owned in the town rose more than sixfold between 1582 and 1702. On a visit to Ipswich at the end of the century, Celia Fiennes was sharply critical of the failure of the citizens to exploit their advantages by not attracting manufacturers, engaging in victualling or providing outward cargoes for the colliers which had brought in coal.[8]

Fiennes's assessment of the economic state of Norwich was a much more favourable one, for she found it to be 'a rich thriveing industrious place'. Yet the city had taken some time to recover from the effects of the plague and smallpox epidemics in the 1660s. Although its population had regained its former size by the early 1670s, further growth during that decade was slow, before a period of rapid expansion marked a return to the rate of increase in numbers that the city had experienced in the early seventeenth century. This was fuelled by immigration that added roughly 400 people each year, including a considerable number of Huguenots. The mid-1660s had been a time of economic stagnation, during which the corporation began to investigate the establishment of a workhouse, a project that was not realised until 1712, and in 1670 Thomas Corie wrote gloomily that 'poverty daily invades us like an armed man'. Nevertheless, the city's worsted weaving industry revived and, as Celia Fiennes saw, by the end of the century Norwich's earlier prosperity had returned.[9]

She was equally impressed by the well-being of Deal, not noticing any remaining effects of the plague, and commenting that the town 'looks like a good thriveing place the buildings new and neate brickwork with gardens'. In contrast, she described Southampton as 'almost forsooke and neglected', although in 1662 the Dutch artist William Schellinks had thought it 'a fine, populous town'. In 1683 its leading citizens attributed the fact that the town 'has been a rich place, but now is quite the contrary' to a number of factors, including the cost of the Civil War, high mortality during the plague, the loss of almost all of its ships during the Anglo-Dutch wars, the decline of its textile trade and a sharp reduction in its trade in French wine. Despite a growing coastal trade, Southampton in the late seventeenth century was perceived to be a town in decline, with the plague a contributory cause. Its population fell from 4,200 to 3,000 between the 1590s and 1690s.[10]

Winchester's experience was rather different. Although the loss of population in the epidemic was barely replaced within ten years, and a despondent corporation described the city in 1670 as being 'never in so low and mean condition as now it is', in fact its economy was reviving. Defoe's summary in the early eighteenth century was that Winchester was 'a place of no trade . . . no manufacture, no navigation', but he did find that it had 'a great deal of good company'. This reflected the city's new role as a social and economic focus for the county gentry, who were high-status consumers, and during the late seventeenth century it had drawn in immigrants, aiding its demographic recovery.[11]

Travellers' descriptions are subjective. A town visited on a market day in fine weather soon after the harvest could present a different impression if seen in gloomy winter conditions when there was little visible economic activity. None the less, reactions to these provincial towns badly affected by the plague in 1665–6, together with supporting evidence, do indicate marked contrasts in the rate of recovery from the epidemic. The extent to which plague alone was instrumental in bringing about change is difficult to assess, but it does seem that it served as a catalyst, causing problems for a community with an economy containing structural weaknesses, while one that was inherently sound or adaptable could recover remarkably quickly. Plague could accelerate decline and perhaps make it a more traumatic process than it would have been if the disease had not struck. A town's ability to repopulate by attracting immigrants provides an indicator of its prosperity, especially against the background of the economic problems of the mid-1660s and, over the longer term, a static national population.

The effects of war and dislocation of trade helped continue the economic recession that had begun in 1664 beyond the end of the Second Dutch War in 1667. While the obstacles to trade and manufacturing were removed with the return of peace, the agrarian economy entered a period of low prices and falling rents. Good harvests, improved communications, increased productivity and a rise in imports were factors in depressing prices, but the plague may have contributed in the short term, by contracting the urban market. Perhaps one-twelfth of urban consumers died in the epidemic, and while rapid repopulation, especially of London, suggests that the loss was quickly made up, it was fuelled by migrants from other communities, including urban ones.[12] If patterns of migration to Norwich, Great Yarmouth and Ipswich after the plague were similar to those in other years, then considerable numbers of their immigrants came from other towns and the textile villages of East Anglia, as well as from agricultural communities. The process did not, therefore, replace the missing consumers by a simple transfer of population from the agricultural sector to the urban one.[13] Furthermore, not all towns recovered rapidly. In the aftermath of the Great Plague suppliers of produce to Ipswich and Southampton were faced with a shrunken market that did not revive. This suggests that plague did indeed

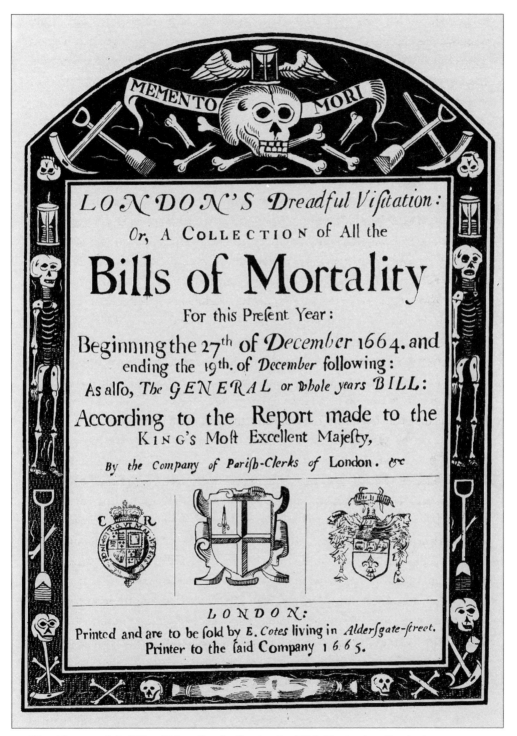

The title page of the Bills of Mortality *for London for 1665.* (Author's collection)

contribute to a situation in which there was an oversupply of agricultural produce, at least in the short term, and hence falling prices. In 1666 and 1667 grain prices were on average two-thirds of those prevailing in 1660–5.[14] But the contribution that plague may have made to the low prices of agricultural produce then or thereafter cannot be separated from other factors, in particular the run of good harvests from 1667 to 1672.

A further cause of the low price levels throughout the 1670s and 1680s was the size of the total domestic market. England's population ceased to grow around 1650 and fell throughout the next three decades, from 5.25 million at the mid-century to 4.9 million in 1680, recovering only slightly during the 1690s, to 5.05 million by 1700.[15] Migration to the larger urban areas, with their high death rates, may have played a part in this, removing from a community its younger, more fertile, members and thus reducing the numbers in their generation having children there. The repopulation of London after the Great Plague was a concentrated phase within a continual process which had an impact on much of southern England, absorbing surplus numbers and depressing the birth rate in those communities supplying the migrants. Graunt observed that 'the great Plague doth not lessen the Inhabitants of the City, but of the Country, who in a short time remove themselves from thence hither'.[16] But while lower levels of fertility may have contributed to the fall in population, the period was one of high mortality rates, with many deaths caused by fevers and smallpox. Fear of smallpox, in particular, seems to have increased during the late seventeenth century. In contrast to plague, it gained the reputation of a disease which struck the wealthier social classes, with Mary II its most notable victim. Although it caused less than 3 per cent of deaths in London in 1629–36, by the early 1680s the proportion was 8 per cent, and an epidemic in the capital was generally followed by more widespread outbreaks in the following year. The incidence of smallpox in Oxford became increasingly common in the 1670s and the 1680s, with virulent outbreaks in 1675 and 1683. Yet Sir William Petty, writing in 1682, still believed that it was plague epidemics in London, occurring on a twenty-year cycle and killing one-fifth of the inhabitants, that checked the growth of national population.[17] Whatever the effects of the Great Plague, the disease could not have had an impact during the late seventeenth century because, unknown to Petty, it had already ceased to be a killer, with the last deaths from plague recorded in the *Bills of Mortality* occurring in 1679, at Rotherhithe.[18] Even so, the column in which plague deaths were entered remained in the *Bills* until 1703, when it was removed.

It may have been because it was the last eruption of the disease that the epidemic of 1665–6 came to be described as 'the Great Plague'. Similar designations had been given to earlier outbreaks, such as that of 1625, which before 1665 was referred to as 'the last great plague'. Certainly, the Great Plague did not have a wide incidence, with fewer than 10 per cent of a sample of 404 parishes across England, but excluding London, recording an unusually high level of mortality. Nevertheless, in urban areas the impact was considerable, with three of the five parishes in Norwich in the sample and seven of the eight in Ipswich recording crisis levels of burials, and overall the mortality rate during 1665-6 was more than 30 per cent above the current level. The sample emphasises both the localised nature of the epidemic and the variation in its impact between regions already noticed, for much of the west of England and parts of the Midlands escaped, while the towns on or near the coasts of East Anglia and the South East were badly affected.[19]

Combining the aggregate for provincial communities where the numbers of plague deaths are known with the figure derived from the London *Bills of Mortality* produces a total of slightly over 100,000 deaths during the Great Plague, or 2 per cent of the population of England. Figures are lacking for only a few of the towns that suffered badly, and so the numbers that are not included in this estimate are largely those from rural parishes. As the disease struck urban areas more severely than rural ones, and the populations of country parishes were such that high mortality levels did not represent large numbers of dead, the estimate is unlikely to excessively under-represent the true figure. Indeed, even if the numbers of non-metropolitan deaths were twice as high as has been allowed for here, the estimated national total would still be no more than approximately 130,000, or the equivalent of 2.5 per cent of the population. In terms of deaths from all causes in the seventeenth and eighteenth centuries the sample of 404 parishes shows eight years with higher mortality than 1665–6, and in a sample of 112 parishes in south-east England the period of the Great Plague does not appear among the fifteen years with most deaths during those centuries.[20] Because of the absence of London from both samples, they undoubtedly give a misleading impression of the impact of the epidemic. Nevertheless, the figures suggest that the designation 'Great Plague' is hardly justified in national terms, certainly in comparison with the scale of mortality in the Black Death.

While the epidemic of 1665–6 was undeniably the 'Great Plague' so far as the inhabitants of Colchester, Southampton, Winchester, Deal, Braintree and Eyam were concerned, the term has generally been applied to London, with its large numbers of plague deaths, rather than to provincial communities. Yet even for

London the description can be questioned, in terms of the proportion of the population who died. Comparison of the levels of mortality is fraught with difficulties because of the uncertainty of the evidence for population size and the allowances that have to be made for those parts of the capital that were added to the *Bills of Mortality*, with nine out-parishes included for the first time during 1603, and Westminster and six other distant parishes in 1636. Graunt sought to overcome the problems by allowing for an increase of 62.5 per cent in the total population between 1625 and 1665. On that basis, and using the peak numbers of weekly burials as an indicator, the plague of 1665 was not as severe as that forty years earlier. In fact, he underestimated the scale of the population increase over the intervening years, and did not compare the total numbers of deaths in the various plague years to examine their relative intensity. When the changes in the population and the expansion in the area within the Bills are allowed for, it is clear that the epidemics in 1563, 1603, 1625 and 1665 saw the highest levels of mortality in the early modern period, and that those in 1578, 1582, 1593 and 1636 were less destructive. The mortality rate in 1563 may have been somewhat higher than in the other most serious outbreaks, and that in 1665 the lowest of the four, although the uncertainties of the evidence, especially for 1563, make definite judgements inappropriate. But if the designation Great Plague were taken to reflect solely the total numbers of deaths, then it would be applied to 1665, which saw more than double the number recorded in 1603 and almost 50 per cent more than in 1625, when the figures are adjusted to allow for the distant parishes.[21]

After the epidemic of the 1660s Thomas Sprat wrote that 'The mortality of this Pestilence exceeded all others of later Ages' and hoped that the reaction would be to spur efforts to prevent future outbreaks of 'this greatest Terror of mankind'. Such epidemics were not attributable to the anger of providence or the cruelty of nature, but to the neglect of mankind in not devising a remedy in the form of an antidote, which surely was within its capabilities.[22] But the medical profession was not able to match Sprat's optimism. Indeed, the agent of plague could not be discovered until the late nineteenth century, following major advances in biological science and microscope optics. What the Great Plague did do was to sharpen the controversy between those who favoured traditional Galenic methods and the champions of Paracelsian medicine, as expounded by the Dutch alchemist Johannes Baptista van Helmont, particularly in his *The Tomb of Plague*, which had been published in English in 1662. The division was so sharp that in 1665 the advocates of Paracelsianism established a Society of Chemical Physicians, in direct challenge to the College of Physicians. But the

Society was short-lived and the debate regarding plague did not – and in the current state of knowledge could not – come close to identifying the cause of the disease and therefore produce effective treatment. What did improve in the late seventeenth century was the standard of medical observation, by Thomas Sydenham and others.[23] Even so, and in contrast to Sprat's confidence, the Dutch physician Paul Barbette, writing in 1676, opined that the plague was beyond human comprehension, and, after considering the nature of the symptoms and various treatments, could do no better than to recommend moving away when an epidemic threatened. Robert Boyle also contributed to the debate, examining the causes and manifestations of plague and concluding that, even though some cures seemed to work in some circumstances, no solution had been found.[24]

With the failure to produce an effective treatment, those which were advocated in the late seventeenth century seem not to have differed greatly in their nature

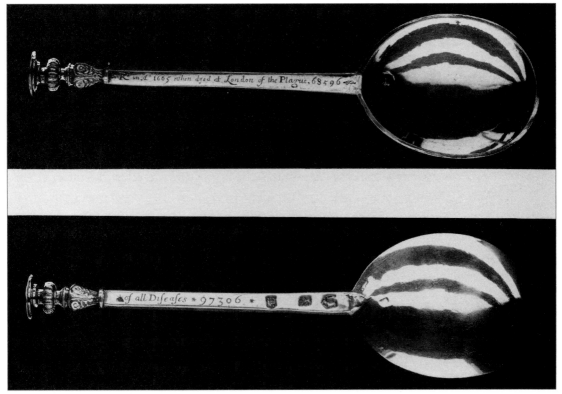

The objects produced in commemoration of the Great Plague include this pewter spoon, which has the figures for deaths in London, taken from the Bills of Mortality. *(© Museum of London)*

from the earlier medicines. In his *The Pharmacopean Physician's Repository* of 1670 Edward Maynwaringe recommended 'bezoardick extract' as an antidote against the plague, claiming that its efficacy had been 'sufficiently proved' during the epidemic of 1665. Nor was lay opinion of the cause of the disease greatly altered after the Great Plague. William Camden, the antiquary, had observed that the conjunction of Saturn and Capricorn coincided with each great plague in London. Recounting this, John Aubrey added that the same conjunction had also occurred in 1625 and again in 1665.[25]

The plague years of the 1660s certainly continued to loom large in the public consciousness, especially when the disease threatened once more. It moved across Flanders and northern France between 1666 and 1668, with epidemics at Dunkirk, Lille, Laon, Beauvais and Rouen. Among the worst affected places were Dieppe and Amiens, which lost between 10 and 20 per cent of their populations, or a similar proportion to the death toll in some English towns during the Great Plague. The authorities imposed strict quarantine measures, and the plague did not reach Paris.[26] A more severe epidemic devastated parts of central Europe in 1679–82, with Buda, Prague and Belgrade badly affected, Graz losing almost a quarter of its inhabitants, and Vienna suffering its highest mortality of the century, with at least 76,000 deaths.[27] Plague also struck Malta in 1675 and southern Spain between 1676 and 1682, prompting the Privy Council to put in place quarantine restrictions on shipping from Malaga.[28] But it was outbreaks in the early eighteenth century in northern Europe and the western Mediterranean that once more raised the spectre of an epidemic in Britain, and led to the adoption of further countermeasures.

The disease, spreading northwards from the Turkish empire, reached Poland in 1708-9, the Baltic in 1710, and Sweden and Denmark before the end of that year. Riga, Tallinn and Königsberg all lost a quarter or more of their inhabitants. A contemporary estimate put the number of deaths in Copenhagen at 25,000 in the space of six months in 1711, and there were 40,000 deaths in Stockholm. But the disease was not confined to the towns, for the rural population of Estonia and Livonia also suffered high rates of mortality.[29] As 10 per cent of imports into England came from Scandinavia and the Baltic lands the epidemic caused considerable, and understandable, alarm. In December 1710 Jonathan Swift wrote that 'We are terribly afraid of the plague', admitting that he had been fearful for the past two years. He had accosted Robert Harley, who was then Chancellor of the Exchequer, and begged him 'for the love of God to take some care about it, or we are all ruined'. Swift's concern reflected the fear that the prospect of a plague epidemic could still arouse, more than forty years after the last outbreak in Britain. In fact, action had already been taken, with orders in 1709 compelling ships from the Baltic to perform quarantine, but Swift thought that vessels were evading it. Anxieties were heightened by a report that the disease had broken out at Newcastle upon Tyne, although that proved to be false. Fears were aroused once more in 1712, when some London physicians became concerned that a fever that was then present was the precursor of the plague, and again in the following year, with the return of soldiers from the continent who were suspected of carrying the disease.[30]

Daniel Defoe referred to the fever as the 'new and unaccountable distemper' in an issue of his periodical the *Review* in August 1712, where he noted that it would 'be mortal, and . . . contagious'. In the following issues he felt the need to defend himself against criticism that he was being alarmist, worrying his readers 'with melancholy notions of the plague'. His defence was that he was countering complacency, for a similar fever had preceded the Great Plague, the plague had been spreading across eastern Europe in recent years and he expected that it would reach Britain in 1713. He also printed the *Bill of Mortality* for London for 12–19 September 1665, the worst week of the epidemic, because 'I think the thing a little too much forgotten amongst us.'[31] Despite his fears and the dangers, the outbreak did not spread to western Europe.

Even more alarming than the fever in 1712 was the epidemic that brought death to the towns of southern France in 1720 and 1721. It began at the end of July 1720 at Marseille, reputedly when two dockers unloading wool from a ship that had come from Sidon were taken ill with bubonic plague. A cordon was quickly put in place around the city, but it had to be moved further away, as the disease spread. By the end of the outbreak roughly 40,000 of the city's 90,000 inhabitants had died, and similarly high levels of mortality were experienced at Toulon, Aix-en-Provence, Apt, Arles and other towns.

In response, in August 1720 the Privy Council directed that no goods or persons from ships coming from the Mediterranean were to be allowed to land, and that the quarantine orders employed in 1710–11 should be renewed. In the Thames estuary, quarantine stations were set up at Standgate Creek on the Medway, Sharpfleet Creek and the lower end of The Hope. The order ruled that some goods, including a wide range of textiles, feathers, wool and hair, could not be landed even on the completion of the forty-day quarantine. Because of trade connections the regulations were soon extended to vessels from ports in the Bay of Biscay, the Channel Islands and the Isle of Man, and from September 1721

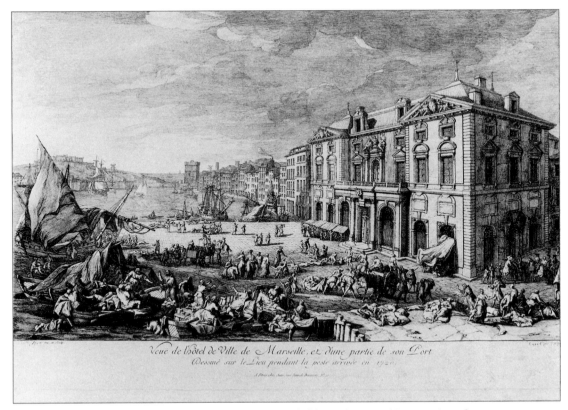

The effects of the plague epidemic at Marseille in 1720 are shown in this engraving after a painting by Michael Serre. (© The Wellcome Institute Library, London)

anyone coming from France north of the Bay of Biscay was required to produce a bill of health before landing, or to serve the period of quarantine.[32]

The government's powers respecting quarantine were reinforced by a further Act of Parliament, and the closure of a possible loophole by which crews of vessels suspected of smuggling could escape inspection. The ship which carried Luigi Marsigli from Livorno reached the Thames in October 1721, and there had to perform quarantine, together with forty other vessels. Indeed, the numerous requests for the release of ships and cargoes from quarantine that came before the Privy Council during the next two years indicate both that the procedures were enforced and the extent of disruption that was caused. Partly to set an example and partly to discourage trade with Turkey, in February 1721 two ships that had been loaded at Cyprus and Scanderoon were burnt, together with their cargoes.[33]

In the autumn of 1721 the Privy Council turned its attention to the steps that should be taken if the plague reached London, although by then the epidemic in Provence was on the wane. Sir Hans Sloane, President of the College of Physicians, and his colleagues Richard Mead and John Arbuthnot were directed to investigate how the information recorded in the *Bills of Mortality* could be improved, in order to obtain 'the earliest and truest Intelligence of the plague, in case it should break out'. The ministers of several of the largest London parishes were questioned regarding the condition of their burial vaults and churchyards, and the parish officers were instructed to make improvements to them. An estimate was obtained of the cost of erecting lazarettos, the corporation of London was consulted about earlier plague regulations, and the Privy Council also received a summary of the steps which had been taken in 1625 and 1665. Orders regarding the keeping of pigs within the metropolis, and the state of several 'stinking Ditches about the Skirts of the Town', provided parallels with the precautions taken during the Great Plague.[34]

The recommendations made by Richard Mead in his *Short Discourse concerning Pestilential Contagion and the Methods to be used to Prevent it* also echoed earlier proposals, especially those made by Sir Theodore de Mayerne in 1631 and the Earl of Craven in 1666. Mead supported the policy of quarantining shipping from areas that were infected and was a further critic of household isolation once the plague had broken out, favouring the separation of the victims from those who had been in contact with them. He also recommended the isolation of towns where the disease was present, with those wishing to pass out through the cordon being subjected to a quarantine period of twenty days. The French government had adopted such a policy, isolating the Provençal towns where plague had broken out. Sir Hans Sloane and his colleagues also submitted a report which owed much to previous practices and the experience gained during the Great Plague. They recommended dividing the metropolis into six health districts and removing the sick to pest-houses around the city, but distinguishing those who were suspected contacts from those who had the disease. The Privy Council also received a report from Sir John Colbatch, outlining steps that could be taken if the plague reached England, especially with regard to the maintenance of order. Aware that in past outbreaks some people had deliberately spread the disease, Colbatch favoured a show of military strength to deal with the disruption which he anticipated, with armed militia in each health district and the quartering of troops near London in case the poor became unruly.[35]

Before the government took action its legal officers were instructed to examine the legality of a ban on trade with a country where plague was suspected, and the crown's powers regarding the granting of commissions of health. They reported that the existing powers were inadequate, and although commissioners of health were appointed in November 1721, the order was rescinded less than three months later.[36] Resistance to some aspects of the policy of isolation had arisen, both within parliament and outside it, fuelled by critical pamphlets and political opponents of the government. The forcible removal of families to pest-houses and the sealing off of infected communities within lines of earthworks were both presented as attacks on English liberties and were equated with the use of 'arbitrary' power, as employed during the epidemic in France. In addition, the need for a policy of quarantining was questioned by those who did not accept that the plague was contagious and brought from places which had the disease, and was opposed by the mercantile sector, headed by the Levant Company. In such a climate it proved to be politically impossible for Sir Robert Walpole, then endeavouring to consolidate his hold on power, not only to strengthen further the Quarantine Act passed in January 1721, but even to maintain the powers which it gave to the government in respect of steps to be taken if the plague reached England. Measures empowering the establishment of commissions of health, *cordons sanitaire* manned by troops around infected towns, with the inhabitants kept within the lines by force if necessary, and the removal of plague victims from their homes, with penalties for non-compliance, could not be supported. Thus, the Quarantine Act of February 1722 repealed those sections of the earlier Act that related to the handling of a domestic epidemic, although retained the policy of quarantining shipping.[37]

The drastic procedures outlined in the Act of 1721 were not revived and indeed were not required, for although plague continued to ravage parts of eastern Europe and the lands around the eastern Mediterranean throughout the eighteenth century, it did not return to western Europe after the outbreak in Provence had come to an end. Despite the absence of plague from western Europe after the early 1720s, there was still a great awareness of the threat of the disease and a continuing debate on the methods that should be taken to combat it. The government took stringent precautions from time to time, when the danger seemed to have increased. Vessels coming from the Levant were required to have a bill of health to show that their cargoes had been opened and aired at one of seven specified lazarettos in the western Mediterranean, and those thought to carry a risk were to serve their period of quarantine in the Scilly

Isles. Smuggling was recognised as a potential threat, but as it was generally carried out in small boats over relatively short distances the danger may have been exaggerated.[38]

Fumigation continued to be the favoured way of disinfecting goods that may have been carrying the plague, and was employed in the lazarettos in the Mediterranean until well into the nineteenth century. Great faith was still placed in the efficacy of strong-smelling herbs. In 1781 the French writer Jean-Jacques Menuret reported how 'immense storerooms' of rue and other drugs had preserved a whole district of London from infection during the Great Plague. It was not only the smell of herbs that was regarded as a protection, however, for the *Encyclopédie méthodique* of 1787 described how all the cesspools in London had been opened in 1665, in the belief that their odour could drive away the plague. As late as the 1790s the medical authorities at Madrid believed that without the stench of sewage that pervaded the city the plague would soon return.[39]

A plague epidemic struck Messina, in Sicily, in 1743, but the disease gradually became a more distant threat, ravaging the Turkish empire and from time to time erupting into Russia, killing 56,672 people in an epidemic in Moscow in 1771.[40] The population of Constantinople endured frequent outbreaks of the disease, including especially severe ones in 1778 and 1813. Yet with the adoption of quarantining, the erection of isolation hospitals and appointment of a sanitary council, after 1836, plague had been almost eradicated from the city by the middle of the nineteenth century.[41] The third International Sanitary Conference was held in Constantinople in 1866, and by then the most serious threat to public health was not plague but cholera, which had spread out from India after 1817, reaching Britain in 1832.

The continuing threat of plague generated much interest outside government and medical circles. The epidemic of the 1660s naturally attracted attention, with additions to the existing literature on the subject, including Nathaniel Hodges's *Loimologia: or, an Historical Account of the Plague in London in 1665*, which appeared in 1720, and *A Collection of very Valuable and Scarce Pieces relating to the last Plague in the Year 1665*, which included the London plague orders and the prescriptions recommended by the College of Physicians. Defoe had returned to the subject in *Memoirs of a Cavalier*, published in 1720. The narrator, a soldier of fortune in the 1630s and 1640s, reported that while in Italy in 1630 he had contracted 'a slow lingring Fever' that developed into the plague. The pain caused by a bubo on his neck made him 'raging mad', but this eased soon after it had burst, and he survived.[42] Defoe also reported the steps taken to limit the spread of

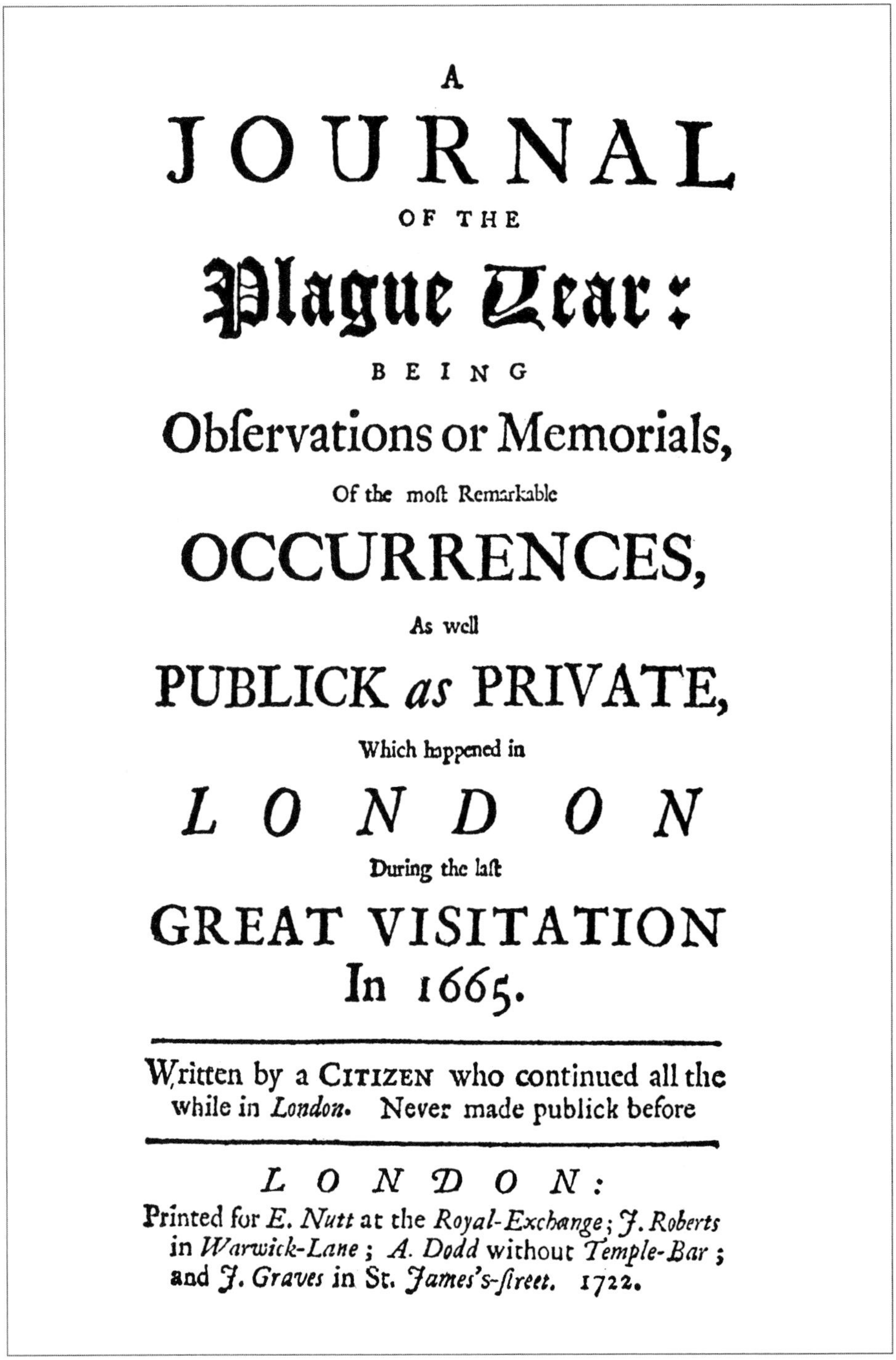

A

JOURNAL

OF THE

𝕻lague 𝖄ear:

B E I N G

Obſervations or Memorials,

Of the moſt Remarkable

OCCURRENCES,

As well

PUBLICK *as* PRIVATE,

Which happened in

L O N D O N

During the laſt

GREAT VISITATION
In 1665.

Written by a CITIZEN who continued all the while in *London.* Never made publick before

L O N D O N :
Printed for *E. Nutt* at the *Royal-Exchange*; *J. Roberts* in *Warwick-Lane*; *A. Dodd* without *Temple-Bar*; and *J. Graves* in St. *James's-ſtreet.* 1722.

The title page of Daniel Defoe's popular novel, A Journal of the Plague Year. (Unknown; courtesy of Penguin)

plague in Provence, including the shooting of those who tried to leave Toulon, and contributed to the debate on the preventive measures that should be taken in Britain.[43] In 1722 he published two books on the plague, *Due Preparations for the Plague, as well for Soul as Body* and *A Journal of the Plague Year*, both of which are set in 1665. The former consists of a set of dialogues in the context of an epidemic on the continent and the fear that it will spread to England, while the latter is an imaginative reconstruction of the plague, written in the first person by 'a Citizen who continued all the while in London', identified only as H.F. The account in *A Journal* is so effective that it led to speculation that Defoe wrote it from memory, and so it could be treated as primary evidence, although he was only five years old in 1665, or that H.F. was his uncle, Henry Foe. Others regarded *A Journal* as a work of pure fiction.[44] In fact, his sources can be identified from contemporary material, a task carried out by Watson Nicholson. Having done that, he was also inclined to accept the authenticity of the anecdotes which are included, believing Defoe to have been overscrupulous in not vouching for their accuracy. Indeed, Nicholson's conclusion was to include the book with 'authentic histories'.[45]

The evidence for conditions in London during the Great Plague was significantly augmented in the early nineteenth century with the publication for the first time of the diaries of John Evelyn and Samuel Pepys. Evelyn's diary appeared in 1818 and was followed in 1825 by selections from that of Pepys. Further editions of the diaries followed and eventually both were published in full. Pepys, in particular, was a brilliant observer, providing a fascinating delineation of the epidemic in London in 1665 and its effects. The availability of his other papers provided further evidence. He recounted an incident in which a family was confined in a house in Gracechurch Street and the father, in an attempt to save his daughter, passed her naked out of a window to a friend, who then took her to Greenwich.[46] This scene caught the imagination of the artist Frank William Topham, whose painting dated 1898, shows the father passing the girl out of the window. Evelyn's diary also had a wide appeal, providing further personal testimony of conditions during the epidemic, as well as material for a range of other subjects. These included the career of the woodcarver and sculptor Grinling Gibbons, who Evelyn first mentioned in 1671. At the time of the plague Gibbons had not yet come to England from Holland, but the temptation to link a well-known figure from the Restoration period with one of its most famous events proved to be irresistible. In *The Carved Cartoon*, published in 1874, the novelist Austin Clare described Gibbons's life in London during the Great Plague, and in

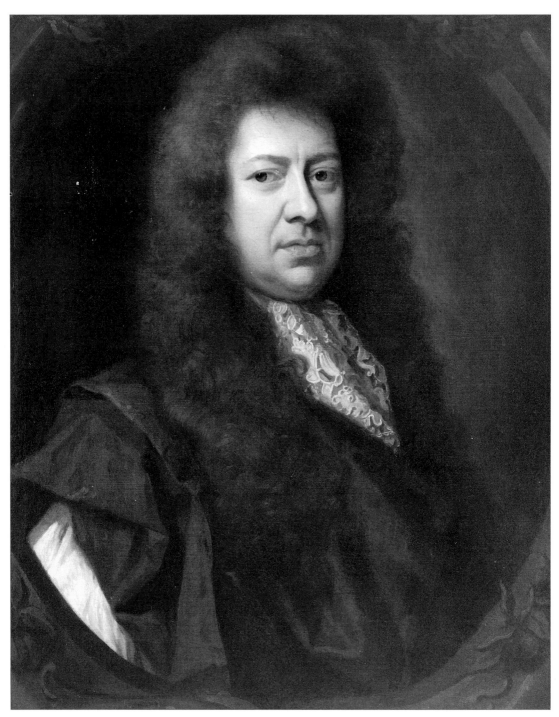

Samuel Pepys, administrator of the Royal Navy and diarist, by Godfrey Kneller. (© National Maritime Museum, Greenwich, London)

1932 the book was adapted as a play for children. A later dramatisation, by Brian Way, also set Gibbons's early life in the capital during the epidemic, and carried the dramatic title *Grinling Gibbons and the Plague of London*.[47]

During the eighteenth century the impact of the Great Plague on provincial communities attracted attention. In *A Tour through the Whole Island of Great Britain*, Defoe gave a figure of 'upwards of 5259' burials at Colchester in 1665 and he commented that the proportional loss was greater even than at London. Detailed work on the numbers of deaths was carried out by the local historian Philip Morant, rector of St Mary-at-the-Walls in the town, who included his findings in *The History and Antiquities of Colchester*, which appeared in 1748.[48] But far greater attention came to be focused on the events at Eyam. Brief accounts were included in Richard Mead's *A Discourse on the Plague* of 1744 and Thomas Short's *A General Chronological History of the Air*, published five years later. Mead drew his information on the way in which the disease had been contained within the parish from the son of William Mompesson, the rector, and 'another worthy Gentleman', although Short did not mention that aspect of the outbreak at all. Other accounts followed in the 1790s and later, but it was William Wood's *The History and Antiquities of Eyam*, which first appeared in 1842, that provided the basis for the parish's fame. Wood based his narrative on the evidence of the parish registers and local oral tradition, and it was drawn upon for later descriptions of the episode and the recognition of the selfless courage of the parishioners, the heroes of Eyam, in refusing to flee and thereby risk spreading the disease. He lavished praise on both the inhabitants and Mompesson, and chiefly because of his account of the epidemic Eyam has become associated with the Great Plague in a way that no other place has, with the exception of London.[49]

From the end of the nineteenth century the available historical evidence had to be reassessed in the light of the identification of the plague bacillus and the means by which the disease was transmitted. The sources for the Great Plague were examined for possible information on rats and their behaviour, but this is small and incidental, for contemporaries had not made the link between the animal and the plague. The evidence consists primarily of the numerical returns of the *Bills of Mortality* and parish registers, and observations by contemporaries that are circumscribed by their perceptions of the cause and spread of plague. The effects on the rat population may have gone unnoticed or unreported because of concerns with human suffering and the practical problems of living through an epidemic. Modern studies of the nature and behaviour of the plague bacillus, rats and fleas provide such information as the temperatures at which the rat's flea is active, but it would be imprudent to assume that such factors have remained unchanged since the seventeenth century. Because direct evidence is lacking explanations are necessarily inferential and open to interpretation.

Even before the role of the rat and its flea, *Xenopsylla cheopis*, had been recognised, there had been a prolonged debate regarding the reasons for the disappearance of plague after the 1670s. This could be more clearly focused once the chain connecting the plague bacterium, *Pastuerella pestis mediaevalis*, fleas, rats and humans was established. That chain had been broken at some point, as it had at the end of the first European pandemic, which ended in the 680s, apart from outbreaks around Narbonne in 694 and in southern Italy in 767.[50]

Among the suggestions advanced for the disappearance of plague in Britain was that the Great Fire of London in September 1666 had wiped out the vestiges of the infection within the devastated area. The idea was attractive both in terms of the chronology of the two disasters and the image of fire as a purifying element. Thus, in the early twentieth century Walter Besant wrote that the fire 'purified the soil', although he was aware that current investigations of the plague in India might lead to the abandonment of the association of the disease with polluted ground in which filth had accumulated over several centuries.[51] In fact, by the time that Besant's work was published the means by which plague was spread had been identified. But the discoveries of the 1890s did not put an end to the theory that the Great Fire was instrumental in the disappearance of plague in the British Isles, simply to an adaptation of it. The notion that now became common was that the rats had been killed or driven out by the conflagration. They did not return in their former numbers because the complete replacement within the burnt area of buildings of timber and thatch by those of brick and tile – materials specified in the building regulations issued after the fire – changed the built environment from one that was congenial to rats to one that was hostile to them. The centre of London had been a focus of the infection in which rats and their fleas were concentrated, and from there the plague periodically erupted and spread to other English towns. Christopher Wills, writing more than ninety years after Besant, could still express the view that the fire was of benefit in 'burning out a canker in the heart of the city'.[52]

London did suffer heavily in outbreaks of plague in the sixteenth and seventeenth centuries, but the eradication of certain conditions in a part of it surely cannot account for the abrupt disappearance of the disease from the whole of the city and the rest of the country, let alone from Britain's continental neighbours. The association of the Great Fire with the ending of plague ignores the fact that only one-fifth of just one city was affected by the fire, that the area burnt was that which had suffered comparatively low levels of mortality in 1665, that the districts with high death tolls were those around the City, where the standards of building were lower than in the centre, and they were not touched by the fire, and that in some epidemics plague was reported in other towns before it affected London. The buildings destroyed in the Great Fire were tiled, thatch having been eradicated much earlier because of the fire risk. While the argument that brick structures were less congenial to rats than timber ones was advanced in the mid-seventeenth century, to claim that they were not colonised by them does scant justice to the resourcefulness of rodents in finding homes in structures erected with a variety of materials. Indeed, buildings continued to be constructed using a substantial amount of structural timberwork within the brick shell, and softwood came into increasing use after the Great Fire. Rodents could exploit the gaps between the materials, and the spaces beneath timber floors provided further accessible passages and nesting sites. They find little difficulty today in establishing themselves in buildings, however strong the materials used.

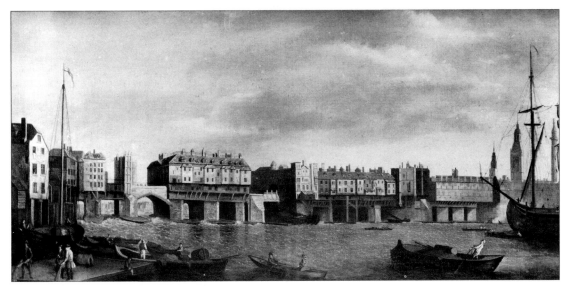

The replacement of timber-and-plaster buildings by those of brick and tile was a gradual process. In this view of London Bridge by Samuel Scott the new brick buildings towards its north end contrast with the older ones at the Southwark end. (© B.T. Batsford Ltd)

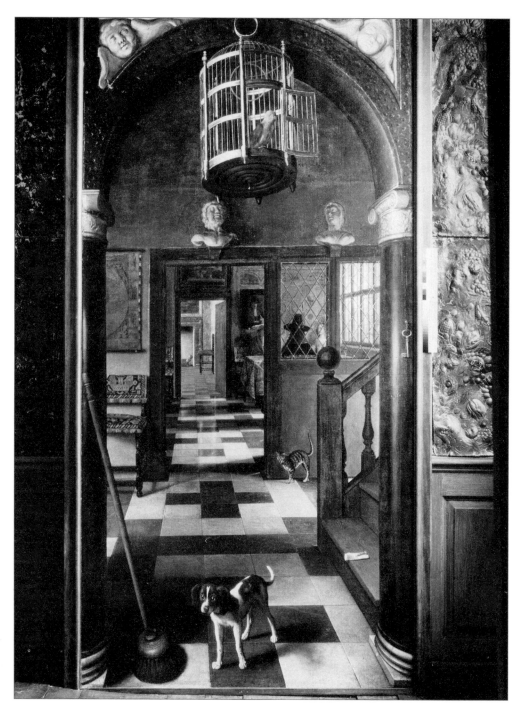

In his View of a Corridor *of 1662 Samuel van Hoogstraten emphasises the cleanliness of the interior with the broom that stands prominently in the foreground. The patrolling dog and cat are further discouragements to rodents.* (© The National Trust/Derrick E. Witty)

In any event, the adoption of brick and tile construction in English towns was a gradual process that was accelerated by major fires in a number of places, but not in many others, and in some regions – notably the south west and East Anglia – it was not completed by the early nineteenth century. Rather than rebuild, some owners chose to add a cladding of external brickwork to the existing structure, to give it an up-to-date appearance and to comply with building regulations. This process changed the exterior, but not those internal elements thought to provide a congenial habitat for rodents.

Perhaps more significant in terms of building practices was the covering of earth floors with stone flags or boards, which, with improved standards of hygiene, may have reduced the extent to which rats and their fleas lived in close proximity to humans. But that closeness was at all times limited by predation by cats and dogs, and changes in flooring and hygiene were gradual processes that varied from region to region, between urban and rural communities, and from one social group to another. Indeed, had such gradual changes to the domestic environment been a major cause of the ending of plague the expected pattern would have been one of a succession of epidemics of diminishing impact, rather than the abrupt end to the disease that did occur.

The outbreaks in the Netherlands in the 1660s show that cleanliness did not confer an immunity from plague. Contemporaries regarded the Dutch preoccupation with cleanliness as being a product of the 'extreme moisture of the air' and consequent danger of disease.[53] The domestic interiors depicted by the painters of the Golden Age are spotless and, even allowing for social bias in the houses portrayed, do not suggest an environment where rats could flourish close to their human occupants. Even in the more disorderly scenes of lower-class life presented by Jan Steen and Adriaen Brouwer cats and dogs are generally present, as they are in the better-off houses. Although such high standards of cleanliness were not characteristic of British houses, this is unlikely to have been a major factor in the absence of plague in the late seventeenth and early eighteenth centuries.

The effect of the weather is uncertain, although it may have played a part. Temperatures during the critical spring and summer months show that although the summers in the late 1660s were particularly warm, the spring months were not. The 1690s was a relatively cool decade, but both the spring and summer periods in the first quarter of the eighteenth century – when the risk of a recurrence of plague was high because of the outbreaks on the continent – saw a recovery of temperatures during those seasons. Generally, spring and summer

The TRUE and EXACT

REPRESENTATION

OF THE

Wonders upon the Water,

During the Last

UNPARALLEL'D FROST

UPON THE

RIVER of *THAMES*, 168¾.

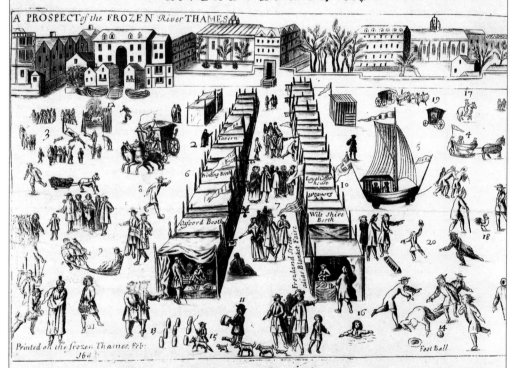

The frost fair on the Thames at London during the winter of 1684. © The Guildhall Library, Corporation of London)

temperatures in England in the late seventeenth and early eighteenth centuries do not indicate a cooling of the climate to the point at which the conditions were not conducive to the breeding of rats' fleas, despite the relatively cool decade of the 1690s. In any case, the epidemics in Scandinavia and the Baltic lands in the early eighteenth century, and in Iceland during the fifteenth, suggest that the plague could be virulent even in cool climates.[54] But although the figures for the winter temperatures in England do not indicate a run of cold seasons, the period did contain the harsh winters of 1684 and 1708/9, with that of 1684 being the coldest in the historical record. It is likely that such severe winters reduced the numbers of rats, as well as their parasites, and that it would have taken some years for them to recover their former numbers.[55]

Whether these two extremely cold winters had a long-term effect on the rat population cannot be determined. However, they are unlikely to have been a contributory cause of the replacement of the black rat, *rattus rattus*, by the brown rat, *rattus norvegicus*, which did not occur until later. In his *Letters from England*, published in 1807, Robert Southey reported that by then the brown rats had 'fairly extirpated the aboriginal ones' and that because they 'came in about the same time as the reigning family, the partisans of the Stuarts used to call them Hanoverians'. His facetious remarks are supported by other evidence that confirms that the success of the brown rat in western Europe occurred in the early eighteenth century, perhaps not until after 1727, when it crossed the River Volga in large numbers, leaving a considerable plague-free interval between the epidemic of the mid-1660s and the demise of the black rat.[56] In fact, this chronology does not support the hypothesis that the change in the rat population helps to explain the disappearance of plague, which was postulated on the basis that the brown rat tends to avoid human habitations, unlike the black one, and that it rarely acts as host for the flea which carries the plague bacillus.

Nor does the experience of the mid-1660s suggest a decline in the virulence of plague at that date, or that the population had developed some resistance to the disease. Indeed, the period following the epidemic, when plague was absent, fitted contemporaries' expectations of the interval between attacks. It may be explained by the high mortality of rats during the Great Plague, so that there were insufficient hosts to disseminate the plague bacillus in the aftermath of the epidemic. This would account for the relatively low mortality in London in 1666, while the disease was having a devastating effect in some towns where both rat and human populations had been unaffected hitherto. The recovery of the rat population should have taken place within a few years, before declining again in the winter of 1684.

Another model that has been suggested for the disappearance of plague in the late seventeenth century is not that the number of rats declined, but that they had developed an immunity to the disease. If that were the case, then the plague ceased to be killer because the infected fleas did not need to leave their hosts and transfer to humans. Without the deaths of the rats, the chain of infection was broken. According to this hypothesis the rats without immunity would have died in the Great Plague, leaving those which had a resistance to the disease. But this had not happened after earlier epidemics, or London, which had been so badly affected, would have had some degree of immunity in 1665.[57] Furthermore, without quarantine new populations of rats susceptible to the disease could have been introduced after an epidemic and caused deaths among the human population. Even if the existing rat population was not numerous enough to support an outbreak on the scale of an epidemic, some deaths from plague surely would have occurred. Despite the weaknesses of this particular interpretation, it may be that a part of the explanation for the disappearance of plague in the seventeenth and eighteenth centuries was some change in the relationship between the plague bacillus, fleas, rats and people that has gone unrecognised, or for which the evidence is not available.

The relative importance of the rat flea and the human flea in the spread of the plague in London is uncertain. It is postulated that as mortality levels rose among the rat population during an epidemic the numbers of rats available to the fleas as hosts fell. The fleas were unable to transfer from the bodies of dead rats to living ones and so moved to humans in their search for warmth, thus spreading the disease. An alternative hypothesis gives less importance to the rat flea, suggesting that, once the epidemic was under way, the principal carrier of plague was the human flea, *Pulex irritans*. Because of the slowness of a black rat moving through an urban environment, and the reluctance of a sick rat to go far from its nest in search of food, it is assumed that in an epidemic which developed gradually and evenly from its source the plague was dispersed by the rat flea. On the other hand, one which spread quickly and erratically is more likely to have been dispersed by the human flea.

The pattern shown by the figures in the weekly London *Bills of Mortality* for 1665 has been examined and, on the basis of the date of the first appearance of plague in a parish, it has been suggested that the pattern of infection was erratic, throwing doubt on the importance of the rat flea in its dissemination, and indeed the role of the rat in the Great Plague. This is supported by the absence from contemporary accounts of reference to dead rats, although they should have been

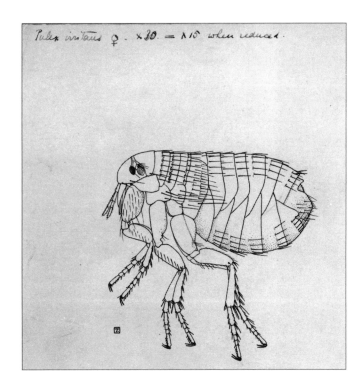

Pulex irritans ♀ . × 80. = ×15 when reduced.

During the debate on the causes of plague epidemics, it has been suggested that the human flea, Pulex irritans, *could have played a part in the dissemination of the disease.* (© The Wellcome Institute Library, London)

dying in such numbers as to have attracted attention. However, the author of another study found that the diffusion of the plague was slow, that it moved steadily from parish to parish, and that had it followed the principal routes crossing the city it would have broken into the intramural area much sooner than it did, suggesting that the disease was carried by rats' fleas.[58] The weakness of the evidence is that the *Bills* record the place of death, not where the victim was infected. Someone who contracted the disease in one parish and subsequently died elsewhere, perhaps some distance away, would be registered in the parish where they died. The first entry for a plague death in a parish is not a sure guide to the distribution or movement of infected rats. It is possible that the disease was carried by rats' fleas that had abandoned their rodent hosts for an alternative warm environment, such as that provided by clothing, other textiles or grain, so that the rat flea was the agent, but the pattern and speed of diffusion reflected human activity.

Over the longer term the imposition and enforcement of effective quarantine measures probably played the greatest part in the eradication of plague from Europe. The implementation of such regulations gradually forced the potential sources of infection eastwards and then south-eastwards. With the adoption by many countries of quarantine as a national policy, not just a local or municipal one, it came to be applied widely, reducing the chance of evasion. Shipping was easier to control than movement overland and so western Europe was freed from plague earlier than the central and eastern parts of the continent, but the countries bordering on the Turkish empire also came to impose effective *cordons sanitaire*.[59] The success of the government's strategy was, therefore, dependent not only on the efficient administration of quarantine at British ports, but also on similar policies being applied stringently by other countries. Thus, the success in preventing the epidemic in Scandinavia and the Baltic in the 1710s from spreading to Britain may have owed as much to strict controls enforced by the authorities in the Netherlands, which carried the bulk of trade with the region, as to those imposed by the British government. It was as well that the plague did not reach Amsterdam, if only because of the many sailings from there to Britain, which made it difficult to intercept all vessels. Similarly, the decisiveness and firmness with which the French government dealt with the epidemic in Provence in the early 1720s contained the disease there, with British controls acting as a secondary line of defence.

As the policy was enforced in those countries trading with the eastern Mediterranean, the risk of the disease being brought from there was greatly reduced. A vessel coming from the Levant to Britain and stopping at an intermediate port would have had to perform a period of quarantine, and the direct voyage would have taken at least twenty-five days. In either case, it is unlikely that the rat's flea could have survived.[60] Of course, this was not known at the time, and it was argued that quarantine was not the reason for the disappearance of the disease from western Europe. The procedures could not be completely secure and trade with the Levant had greatly increased after the 1660s, yet the plague, still rife in its ports, had not spread to western Europe. Smyrna experienced nine epidemics between 1713 and 1792, and in only twenty years during that period was it plague-free, but shipping from there had not brought the disease.[61] It could also have been objected that quarantine had failed to save England in 1665 and that there had been other spectacular failures of the policy from time to time. Although regulations in Italy were deemed to be especially strict, in the 1650s they had not prevented very destructive outbreaks of plague in a number of cities in different regions. Nor had the uncompromising measures taken to contain the plague in Provence in the early 1720s been successful in preventing its spread beyond Marseille, despite the cordon

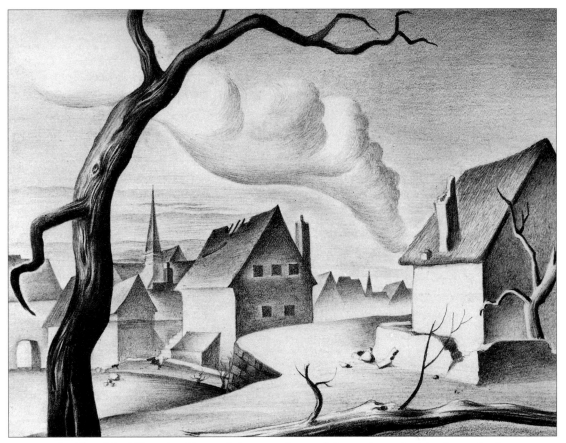

In Albert Lloyd Tartar's mid-twentieth century image of plague, the smoke rising from a desolate town signifies the beginnings of an epidemic. (© The Wellcome Institute Library, London)

established around the city. Moreover, the contagiousness of the disease was not universally accepted and its incidence continued to be ascribed to local conditions and the effects of miasma. The debate between the contagionists and the anti-contagionists attracted considerable professional and lay attention, with the anti-contagionists' views gaining much ground by the middle of the nineteenth century. In addition to doubts about the way in which plague was disseminated, there were also mercantile objections to the policy of quarantine, because it interrupted trade, and political ones such as those faced by Walpole in the 1720s, relating to what were seen as excessive powers being taken by the government.

With the isolation of the plague bacillus and the realisation of the role of the rat's flea, the policy of quarantining appeared to have been justified and the anticontagionist case disproved. Yet knowledge of the nature of the disease and the way in which it was spread, and a long-established British policy for restricting its diffusion, based on quarantine and isolation, could not prevent the deaths of 12.6 million plague victims in India between 1898 and 1948. During this third pandemic plague deaths occurred at Cardiff in 1900 and 1901, Liverpool in 1901 and 1914, and, a more doubtful diagnosis, in Suffolk in 1910, but no widespread outbreak followed.[62]

Thus, the Great Plague of 1665–6 remains the last bubonic plague epidemic in Britain. Although not commemorated by a stone pillar, as is the Great Fire of London, or by a column such as that erected in Vienna after the plague of 1679–80, it is one of the best-known occurrences in British history. This may be due in part to its literary heritage, especially the enduring popularity of Defoe's *A Journal of the Plague Year* and the perceptive account in Pepys's diary, and perhaps to the fact that the Great Fire occurred so soon after the plague had caused such high mortality in London, fixing the mid-1660s as a period of dramatic disasters. The physical manifestations of plague and the high levels of mortality among those infected made it one of the most feared of diseases, attracting attention in a way that other large-scale killers, such as influenza, did not. Discussing the response to an outbreak of plague, in 1766 Murdoch Mackenzie wrote that it was 'a great preservative to be under no apprehension, and to guard as much as possible against dismal thoughts and imaginations upon such occasions'.[63] Even a hundred years after the Great Plague, few would have found it easy to follow such sanguine advice.

Notes

1. Plague and Society

1.   R. Horrox (ed.), *The Black Death* (Manchester, Manchester University Press, 1994), p. 76.

2.   C. Platt, *King Death. The Black Death and its aftermath in late-medieval England* (London, UCL Press, 1996), pp. 100–3.

3.   Thomas More, *Utopia* (London, Dent, 1994), p. 70.

4.   P. Ziegler, *The Black Death* (Harmondsworth, Penguin, 1970), p. 51.

5.   P. Slack, *The Impact of Plague in Tudor and Stuart England* (London, Routledge & Kegan Paul, 1985), p. 43.

6.   Ziegler, *Black Death*, pp. 20–2, 37–9; Benedetto Bonfigli, 'Gonfalone di San Franceso al Prato', 1464; Gonfalone, Santa Maria Nuova, Perugia, 1471.

7.   K. Thomas, *Religion and the Decline of Magic* (Harmondsworth, Penguin, 1973), pp. 91–102, 667–8.

8.   V.T. Sternberg, 'Predictions of the Fire and Plague of London', *Notes and Queries*, 1st series, 7 (1853), 80.

9.   Thomas, *Religion*, p. 388.

10. W. Gouge, *God's Three Arrows* (1631), cited in Thomas, *Religion*, p. 790.

11. B. Pullan, 'Plague and perceptions of the poor in early modern Italy', in T. Ranger and P. Slack (eds), *Epidemics and ideas: Essays on the historical perception of pestilence* (Cambridge, Cambridge University Press, 1992), pp. 107–11; C.M. Cipolla, 'The Plague and the Pre-Malthus Malthusians', *Journal of European Economic History*, 3 (1974), 277–84.

12. W.H. McNeill, *Plagues and Peoples* (New York, Doubleday, 1989), p. 151; C.M. Cipolla, *Public Health and the Medical Profession in the Renaissance* (Cambridge, Cambridge University Press, 1976), p. 29.

13. H. Ballon, *The Paris of Henri IV: Architecture and Urbanism* (Cambridge, Mass., MIT Press, 1991), p. 175; E.S. de Beer (ed.), *The Diary of John Evelyn* (London, Oxford University Press, 1959), p. 250.

14. C.M. Cipolla, *Fighting the Plague in Seventeenth-Century Italy* (Madison, University of Wisconsin Press, 1981), pp. 39–41.

15. Cipolla, *Public Health*, pp. 7–18.

16. Cipolla, *Public Health*, p. 31.

17. HMC, *Fifteenth Report, appendix: Manuscripts of J.M. Heathcote* (London, HMSO, 1899), p. 213.

18. G. Rosen, *A History of Public Health* (Baltimore and London, John Hopkins University Press, 1993), p. 45; Cipolla, *Public Health*, p. 18.

19. J. Israel, *The Dutch Republic: Its Rise, Greatness, and Fall, 1477–1806* (Oxford, Clarendon Press, 1995), p. 329; P. Zumthor, *Daily Life in Rembrandt's Holland* (Stanford, Stanford University Press, 1994), pp. 149, 155.

20. D. Haks and M.C. van der Sman (eds), *Dutch Society in the Age of Vermeer* (Zwolle, Waanders, 1996), pp. 42, 44, 64, 67.

21. E. Le Roy Ladurie, *The Peasants of Languedoc* (Urbana, University of Illinois Press, 1976), p. 141; R.S. Duplessis, *Lille and the Dutch Revolt: Urban Stability in an Era of Revolution 1500–1582* (Cambridge, Cambridge University Press, 1991), pp. 148, 253.

22. Ballon, *Paris*, pp. 172–95; O. Ranum, *Paris in the Age of Absolutism* (New York, John Wiley, 1968), p. 80.

23. J.R. Maddicot, 'Plague in Seventh-Century England', *Past and Present*, 156 (1997), 9–54; J. Hatcher, *Plague, Population and the English Economy 1348–1530* (London, Macmillan, 1977), reprinted in M. Anderson (ed.), *British population history from the Black Death to the present day* (Cambridge, Cambridge University Press, 1996), p. 30.

24. Hatcher, *Plague, Population and the English Economy*, pp. 21–2, 63–4; Platt, *King Death*, pp. 20–1, 33–5.

25. VCH, *Gloucestershire*, vol. 4 (London, 1988), p. 74; Slack, *Impact of Plague*, pp. 61–3.

26. Slack, *Impact of Plague*, p. 90.

27. Slack, *Impact of Plague*, pp. 201–2.

28. Slack, *Impact of Plague*, pp. 203–4; J.H. Thomas, *Town Government in the Sixteenth Century* (London, Allen & Unwin, 1933, reprinted New York, Kelley, 1969), p. 151.

29. P. Slack, 'Metropolitan government in crisis: the response to plague', in A.L. Beier and R. Finlay (eds), *London 1500–1700: The making of the metropolis* (London, Longman, 1986), p. 69.

30. M.S.R. Jenner, 'The Great Dog Massacre', in W.G. Naphy and P. Roberts (eds), *Fear in early modern society* (Manchester, University of Manchester Press, 1997), pp. 47–9, 56.

31. F.P. Wilson, *The Plague in Shakespeare's London* (Oxford, Clarendon Press, 1927), pp. 189–204.

32. R. Finlay and B. Shearer, 'Population growth and suburban expansion', in Beier and Finlay (eds), *London 1500–1700*, pp. 40–9; V. Harding, 'The Population of London, 1550–1700: a review of the published evidence', *The London Journal*, 15 (1990), 112, 114.

33. J.F. Larkin and P.L. Hughes (eds), *Stuart Royal Proclamations Volume I: Royal Proclamations of King James I 1603–1625* (Oxford, Oxford University Press, 1973), pp. 47–8, 398–400.

34. Wilson, *Plague in Shakespeare's London*, pp. 15–16; Slack, *Impact of Plague*, p. 205 and 'Metropolitan government in crisis', pp. 65–7.

35. Slack, *Impact of Plague*, pp. 209–11.

36. Slack, 'Metropolitan government in crisis', pp. 66–7.

37. Wilson, *Plague in Shakespeare's London*, pp. 76–80; W.G. Bell, *The Great Plague in London* (London, Bodley Head, 1924, reprinted London, Bracken Books, 1994), p. 47.

38. Larkin and Hughes (eds), *Stuart Royal Proclamations Volume I*, pp. 164, 238, 251; Slack, *Impact of Plague*, p. 208.

39. E. Gillett and K.A. MacMahon, *A History of Hull* (Hull, Hull University Press, 1985), p. 110.

40. Wilson, *Plague in Shakespeare's London*, pp. 8–9; John Evelyn, *Fumifugium* (1661), reprinted in G. de la Bédoyère (ed.), *The Writings of John Evelyn* (Woodbridge, Boydell Press, 1995), pp. 154–6.

41. S.P. Cerasano, 'Edward Alleyn: 1566–1622', in A. Reid and R. Maniura (eds), *Edward Alleyn: Elizabethan Actor, Jacobean Gentleman* (London, Dulwich Picture Gallery, 1994), p. 15; HMC, *Sixth Report, Manuscripts of the Duke of Northumberland* (London, HMSO, 1877), p. 229.

42. Slack, *Impact of Plague*, pp. 217–19; PRO, SP16/533/17.

43. J.F. Larkin (ed.), *Stuart Royal Proclamations Volume II: Royal Proclamations of King Charles I 1625–1646* (Oxford, Oxford University Press, 1983), pp. 486–7.

44. P. Borsay, *The English Urban Renaissance: Culture and Society in the Provincial Town, 1660–1770* (Oxford, Clarendon Press, 1989), pp. 69–70.

45. H[ugh] P[eter], *Good Work for a Good Magistrate* (London, 1651), p. 105; 14 Chas. II, c.2.

46. James Howel, *Londinopolis* (1658), pp. 391–2, 394.

47. B. Cunliffe, *The City of Bath* (Stroud, Sutton, 1986), pp. 108–9.

48. C. Morris (ed.), *The Illustrated Journeys of Celia Fiennes 1685–c. 1712* (Stroud, Sutton, 1995), pp. 73, 136.

49. Thomas, *Religion*, p. 11; Jenner, 'Great Dog Massacre', pp. 47–8; C. Wills, *Plagues: Their Origins, History and Future* (London, HarperCollins, 1996), pp. 72–5.

50. L. Bradley, 'Some Medical Aspects of Plague', in *The Plague Reconsidered: A new look at its origins and effects in 16th and 17th Century England* (Matlock, Local Population Studies Supplement, 1977), pp. 12–14.

51. Cipolla, *Fighting the Plague*, pp. 9–13, 99.

52. LMA, acc.1876/AR/3/20A; J.A.I. Champion, *London's Dreaded Visitation. The Social Geography of the Great Plague in 1665* (London, Historical Geography Research Series, 31, 1995), p. 8.

53. *Acts of the Privy Council, 1630–1631* (London, HMSO, 1964), p. 92.

54. Slack, *Impact of Plague*, pp. 148–9, 239; J.C. Robertson, 'Reckoning with London: interpreting the *Bills of Mortality* before John Graunt', *Urban History*, 23 (1996), 325–50; *William Whiteway of Dorchester His Diary 1618 to 1635* (Dorset Record Society, vol. 12, 1991), p. 110.

55. Slack, *Impact of Plague*, pp. 257–62, 269.

56. B. Frith, 'Some aspects of the history of medicine in Gloucestershire, 1500–1800', *Transactions of the Bristol and Gloucestershire Archaeological Society*, 108 (1990), 9.

57. *William Whiteway His Diary*, pp. 83–4, 86.

58. Larkin (ed.), *Stuart Royal Proclamations Volume II*, pp. 85, 98.

59. Slack, *Impact of Plague*, pp. 237, 243.

60. Cipolla, *Public Health*, p. 57; J.C. Brown, *In the Shadow of Florence: Provincial Society in Renaissance Pescia* (Oxford, Oxford University Press, 1982), pp. 56–8; G. Parker, *The Army of Flanders and the Spanish Road 1567–1659* (Cambridge, Cambridge University Press), 1972, p. 43 and *Europe in Crisis, 1598–1640* (Brighton, Harvester, 1980), pp. 23–5, 288.

61. *CSPVen*, 1640–2, p. 207.

62. J. Stoye, *English Travellers Abroad, 1604–1667* (2nd edn, London and New Haven, Yale University Press, 1989), pp. 94, 123, 294.

63. W.H.D. Longstaffe (ed.), *Memoirs of the Life of Mr. Ambrose Barnes* (vol. 50, Surtees Society, 1867), p. 43; H. Roseveare (ed.), *Markets and Merchants of the Late Seventeenth Century: The Marescoe-David Letters, 1668–1680* (London, British Academy, Records of Social and Economic History, new series, 12, 1987), pp. 87–8.

64. A.D. Dyer, *The City of Worcester in the sixteenth century* (Leicester, Leicester University Press, 1973), pp. 21–2, 44–6; Slack, *Impact of Plague*, pp. 62, 102–4.

65. I. Roy, 'England turned Germany? The Aftermath of the Civil War in its European Context', *Transactions of the Royal Historical Society*, 5th series, 28 (1978), 142 and 'The city of Oxford, 1640–60' in R.C. Richardson (ed.), *Town and Countryside in the English Revolution* (Manchester, Manchester University Press, 1992), p. 151.

66. RCHME, *Newark on Trent, the Civil War Siegeworks* (London, HMSO, 1964), pp. 23–4.

67. P. Tennant, *The Civil War in Stratford-upon-Avon. Conflict and Community in South Warwickshire, 1642–1646* (Stroud, Sutton, 1996), p. 125; N.C. Oswald, 'Epidemics in Devon, 1538–1837', *Transactions of the Devonshire Association*, 109 (1977), 94.

68. C. Carlton, *Going to the Wars. The Experience of the British Civil Wars, 1638–1651* (London, Routledge, 1992), pp. 209–10.

69. Slack, *Impact of Plague*, p. 221.

70. The 5th edn is included in C.H. Hull (ed.), *The Economic Writings of Sir William Petty*, (2 vols, Cambridge, Cambridge University Press, 1899), vol. 2, pp. 315–435.

71. Howel, *Londinopolis*, p. 389.

72. Hull (ed.), *Economic Writings* vol. 2, p. 366.

2. The Great Plague in London

1.   Israel, *Dutch Republic*, p. 625.

2.   Slack, *Impact of Plague*, p. 222.

3.   Bell, *Great Plague*, p. 14.

4.   G. Manley, 'Central England temperatures: monthly means 1659 to 1973', *Quarterly Journal of the Royal Meteorological Society*, 100 (1974), 393; H.H. Lamb, *Climate: Present, Past and Future* (2 vols, London, Methuen, 1972–7), vol. 2, p. 568; *Diary of Evelyn*, p. 469; R.C. Latham and W. Matthews (eds), *The Diary of Samuel Pepys* (11 vols, London, Bell & Hyman,

1970–83), vol. 5, pp. 355–9; vol. 6, pp. 32, 66–7; W. Nicholson, *The Historical Sources of Defoe's Journal of the Plague Year* (Boston, Mass., Stratford, 1919), p. 153; BL, Add. MS 10,117, f. 131.

5. Hodges, *Loimologia*, in Nicholson, *Historical Sources*, p. 103.

6. The *Bills of Mortality* are in John Bell, *London's Remembrancer: or, A true Accompt of every particular Weeks Christnings and Mortality In all the Years of Pestilence . . .* (1665).

7. G. Huehns (ed.), Edward Hyde, Earl of Clarendon, *Selections from The History of the Rebellion and The Life by Himself* (Oxford, Oxford University Press, 1978), p. 410; *Diary of Pepys*, vol. 6, pp. 110–11; Bell, *Great Plague*, p. 40.

8. Bell, *Great Plague*, p. 19; W.D. Cooper, 'Notices of the last Great Plague, 1665–6; from the Letters of John Allin to Philip Fryth and Samuel Jeake', *Archaeologia*, 37 (1857), 5.

9. *CSPVen*, 1664–6, pp. 151, 182.

10. *CSPVen*, 1664–6, pp. 175, 194–5, 199.

11. Hull (ed.), *Economic Writings*, vol. 2, pp. 356–7; *Diary of Pepys*, vol. 6, pp. 206–7.

12. Hull (ed.), *Economic Writings*, vol. 1, p. 109.

13. HMC, *Tenth Report, Appendix IV, Manuscripts of Captain Stewart* (London, HMSO, 1885), p. 111.

14. BL, Add. MS 10,117, ff. 139–40.

15. S. Porter, 'Death and burial in a London parish: St Mary Woolnoth 1653–99', *The London Journal*, 8 (1982), 79.

16. *Diary of Evelyn*, pp. 476–7.

17. Bell, *Great Plague*, pp. 30, 38.

18. PRO, PC2/58, p. 187.

19. *Diary of Pepys*, vol. 6, pp. 120, 130–1.

20. William Boghurst, *Loimographia*, in Nicholson, *Historical Sources*, p. 126.

21. C.F. Mullett, *The Bubonic Plague and England* (Lexington, University of Kentucky Press, 1956), p. 196; Hodges, *Loimologia*, in Nicholson, *Historical Sources*, p. 101; C. Morris, 'The Plague', in *Diary of Pepys*, vol. 10, p. 330.

22. *Diary of Pepys*, vol. 6, pp. 106, 120; *CSPVen*, 1664–6, p. 142.

23. Champion, *London's Dreaded Visitation*, pp. 8–9; Hodges, *Loimologia*, in Nicholson, *Historical Sources*, p. 107.

24. William Boghurst, *Loimographia*, in Nicholson, *Historical Sources*, pp. 125–6; Richard Baxter, *Reliquiae Baxterianae*, in Bell, *Great Plague*, p. 15; *Diary of Pepys*, vol. 6, pp. 86–7.

25. *Diary of Pepys*, vol. 6, p. 132.

26. *Diary of Pepys*, vol. 6, pp. 128–30, 142; *CSPVen*, 1664–6, p. 182.

27. Bell, *Great Plague*, p. 60; G.P. Elliott (ed.), 'Autobiography and Anecdotes by William Taswell, D.D.', *Camden Miscellany*, vol. 2 (1853), p. 9.

28. *Diary of Pepys*, vol. 6, p. 133.

29. Bell, *Great Plague*, pp. 80–1.

30. *Diary of Pepys*, vol. 6, pp. 133–4, 147–9, 170, 174; N.H. Keble and G.F. Nuttall, *Calendar of the Correspondence of Richard Baxter, Volume II 1660–1696* (Oxford, Oxford University Press, 1991), p. 47.

31. *Diary of Evelyn*, p. 480.

32. A.R. and M.B. Hall (eds.), *The Correspondence of Henry Oldenburg* (13 vols, Madison, University of Wisconsin Press, 1965–86), vol. 2, pp. 430, 449, 479.

33. LMA, acc.262/43/51,63; Cooper, 'Notices of the last Great Plague', p. 6; D. Gardiner (ed.), *The Oxinden and Peyton Letters 1642–1670* (London, Sheldon Press, 1937), p. 306.

34. *Diary of Pepys*, vol. 6, pp. 145, 150, 164, 187–8, 192, 207, 210, 225, 253, 256, 307; vol. 7, p. 30; R.G. Howarth (ed.), *Letters and the Second Diary of Samuel Pepys* (London, Dent, 1933), pp. 24–5.

35. *Diary of Pepys*, vol. 6, pp. 145, 164, 177–8, 187–8, 191, 246, 342; Morris, 'The Plague', pp. 332–5.

36. Nicholson, *Historical Sources*, pp. 154, 156–64.

37. Nicholson, *Historical Sources*, p. 154.

38. *Diary of Pepys*, vol. 6, pp. 174–5, 201; *Diary of Evelyn*, p. 480; Nicholson, *Historical Sources*, pp. 158–9.

39. 'Autobiography and Anecdotes by William Taswell', p. 9.

40. Nicholson, *Historical Sources*, p. 157.

41. J.F.D. Shrewsbury, *A History of Bubonic Plague in the British Isles* (Cambridge, Cambridge University Press, 1970), pp. 479–80.

42. Thomas Vincent, *God's Terrible Voice in the City*, in Nicholson, *Historical Sources*, p. 118; *Diary of Pepys*, vol. 6, p. 120.

43. Bell, *Great Plague*, pp. 96–7.

44. Slack, *Impact of Plague*, p. 246; Charterhouse Muniments, Assembly Orders, C, f. 67.

45. Nicholson, *Historical Sources*, pp. 126–7, 154; *Diary of Pepys*, vol. 6, p. 268.

46. Hodges, *Loimologia*, in Nicholson, *Historical Sources*, p. 111; Bell, *Great Plague*, pp. 38–9, 161.

47. J.G.L. Burnby, *A Study of the English Apothecary from 1660 to 1760* (London, *Medical History*, Supplement No. 3, 1983), pp. 3–4, 7–8, 17–18.

48. Burnby, *English Apothecary*, p. 99.

49. Slack, *Impact of Plague*, p. 244; *Correspondence of Henry Oldenburg*, vol. 2, pp. 483–4.

50. Cooper, 'Notices of the last Great Plague', p. 6.

51. Slack, *Impact of Plague*, p. 245; Nicholson, *Historical Sources*, p. 157; *Diary of Pepys*, vol. 6, p. 155.

52. Bell, *Great Plague*, pp. 99, 259; Hull (ed.), *Economic Writings*, vol. 2, pp. 356–7.

53. Bell, *Great Plague*, p. 51.

54. Bell, *Great Plague*, p. 102; Cooper, 'Notices of the last Great Plague', p. 6.

55. Mullett, *Bubonic Plague and England*, pp. 197–8, 219.

56. Slack, *Impact of Plague*, p. 245; Mullett, *Bubonic Plague and England*, p. 200; Bell, *Great Plague*, p. 35.

57. M.J. Dobson, *Contours of death and disease in early modern England* (Cambridge, Cambridge University Press, 1997), p. 29; Cooper, 'Notices of the last Great Plague', p. 6; Nicholson, *Historical Sources*, pp. 146, 149; *CSPD*, 1664–5, p. 517.

58. *Diary of Pepys*, vol. 6, p. 214; Bodl., MS Add. c.303, ff. 104, 110.

59. Bell, *Great Plague*, pp. 237–8; *Diary of Pepys*, vol. 6, pp. 189, 213, 217; Shrewsbury, *History of Bubonic Plague*, pp. 461, 466; Manley, 'Central England temperatures', p. 393.

60. Bodl., MS Add. c. 303, f. 126.

61. Bell, *Great Plague*, pp. 38–9, 86–8, 160–1, 335–8; Nicholson, *Historical Sources*, p. 112; *Diary of Pepys*, vol. 7, p. 21.

62. W.H. Godfrey, *The Church of Saint Bride, Fleet Street* (London, Survey of London, Monograph No. 15, 1944), p. 29; *Diary of Evelyn*, p. 482.

63. Nicholson, *Historical Sources*, p. 143; R. Hutton, *The Restoration. A Political and Religious History of England and Wales 1658–1667* (Oxford, Oxford University Press, 1985), pp. 232–3.

64. Nicholson, *Historical Sources*, pp. 122, 143, 154; Bell, *Great Plague*, pp. 150–1, 225; Gilbert Burnet, *History of His Own Time* (London, Dent, 1991), p. 79.

65. Bell, *Great Plague*, p. 133; Hutton, *The Restoration*, p. 226.

66. Nicholson, *Historical Sources*, p. 142.

67. Bell, *Great Plague*, p. 197; *CSPD*, 1665–6, p. 107.

68. Nicholson, *Historical Sources*, pp. 146, 154; G.S. Thomson, *Life in a Noble Household* (London, Cape, 1937), p. 361; LMA, acc.262/43/60,66; Slack, *Impact of Plague*, p. 282.

69. Bell, *Great Plague*, pp. 130, 196–7.

70. Slack, 'Metropolitan government in crisis', p. 72; Bell, *Great Plague*, pp. 196–7, 288–9.

71. Lambeth Palace Library, Sheldon's Register, f. 207.

72. J. Champion, 'Epidemics and the built environment in 1665', in J.A.I. Champion (ed.), *Epidemic Disease in London* (London, Centre for Metropolitan History, Working Paper Series no. 1, 1993), p. 48.

73. *Diary of Pepys*, vol. 6, p. 224; Nicholson, *Historical Sources*, pp. 120, 132–3, 146, 162.

74. Nicholson, *Historical Sources*, pp. 35, 104–5, 135.

75. Bell, *Great Plague*, p. 131; Bodl., MS Add. c.303, f. 112.

76. Nicholson, *Historical Sources*, pp. 37–8; *Diary of Pepys*, vol. 6, pp. 207, 211, 213–14; vol. 7, pp. 40–1; C. Gittings, *Death, Burial and the Individual in Early Modern England* (London, Routledge, 1984), p. 78.

77. *Diary of Pepys*, vol. 6, pp. 279, 297.

78. *Diary of Evelyn*, p. 481.

79. 'Autobiography and Anecdotes by William Taswell', p. 9.

80. Harding, 'Burial of the plague dead in early modern London' in Champion (ed.), *Epidemic Disease*, pp. 55–61; '"And one more may be laid there": the Location of Burials in Early Modern London', *The London Journal*, 14 (1989), 120; *Diary of Pepys*, vol. 7, p. 30.

81. BL, Add. MS 10, 117, f. 147.

82. Harding, 'Burial of the plague dead', p. 57; Godfrey, *Church of St Bride*, p. 29; A. Plummer, *The London Weavers' Company 1600–1970* (London, Routledge & Kegan Paul, 1972), p. 189.

83. J.L. Chester (ed.), *The Parish Registers of St. Thomas the Apostle, London . . . 1558 to 1754* (London, Harleian Society, Parish Registers, vol. VI, 1881), pp. 125–38.

84. *Diary of Evelyn*, pp. 479–80.

85. BL, Add. MS 10,117, f. 147; Cooper, 'Notices of the last Great Plague', p. 9.

86. *Correspondence of Henry Oldenburg*, vol. 2, p. 479.

87. Nicholson, *Historical Sources*, pp. 121, 146–7, 149, 158–9; Morris, 'The Plague', p. 332; *Diary of Pepys*, vol. 6, p. 186.

88. 'Autobiography and Anecdotes by William Taswell', p. 10.

89. Champion, *London's Dreaded Visitation*, pp. 82–4; 'Epidemics and the built environment', p. 48.

90. 'Autobiography and Anecdotes by William Taswell', p. 10.

91. *Diary of Pepys*, vol. 6, pp. 207, 268; Shrewsbury, *History of Bubonic Plague*, pp. 479–80.

92. Nicholson, *Historical Sources*, p. 161.

93. *Diary of Pepys*, vol. 6, p. 165.

94. Bell, *Great Plague*, pp. 127, 255; J.N. Biraben, 'Current Medical and Epidemiological Views on Plague', in *The Plague Reconsidered*, p. 27; Cooper, 'Notices of the last Great Plague', p. 9.

95. Morris, 'The Plague', p. 331.

96. Shrewsbury, *History of Bubonic Plague*, p. 476; Champion, *London's Dreaded Visitation*, pp. 108–9.

97. *Diary of Pepys*, vol. 6, pp. 284, 295.

98. BL, Add. MS 10,117, f. 143; Nicholson, *Historical Sources*, p. 163; *Diary of Pepys*, vol. 6, p. 306.

99. Champion, *London's Dreaded Visitation*, pp. 109, 111.

100. J. Spurr, *The Restoration Church of England, 1646–1689* (London and New Haven, Yale University Press, 1991), p. 53; Nicholson, *Historical Sources*, pp. 163–4.

101. PRO, SP29/126/44; J. Spurr, '"Virtue, Religion and Government": the Anglican Uses of Providence', in T. Harris, P. Seaward and M. Goldie (eds), *The Politics of Religion in Restoration England* (Oxford, Blackwell, 1990), pp. 35, 45 n.49.

102. Hutton, *The Restoration*, pp. 230–1; Bell, *Great Plague*, pp. 165, 217–18.

103. *Diary of Evelyn*, pp. 479–85.

104. LMA, acc.262/43/48,49,51,55,58,60,63,71,79.

105. *Diary of Pepys*, vol. 7, p. 35; CLRO, Lord Mayor's Waiting Book, 2, 2 March 1666.

106. *Diary of Pepys*, vol. 6, pp. 335, 337, 340–2; vol. 7, pp. 14, 17; *Diary of Evelyn*, p. 485;. Keble and Nuttall, *Correspondence of Richard Baxter*, Volume II, p. 47; Bell, *Great Plague*, pp. 309–10.

107. Bell, *Great Plague*, p. 321.

108. Clarendon, *Selections*, p. 412; I. Sutherland, 'When was the Great Plague? Mortality in London, 1563 to 1665' in D.V. Glass and R. Revelle (eds), *Population and Social Change* (London, Arnold, 1972), p. 309; Harding, 'Population of London', p. 120; Champion, *London's Dreaded Visitation*, pp. 37–9.

109. Champion, *London's Dreaded Visitation*, pp. 23–9, 40–1; Bell, *Great Plague*, pp. 179–81; CLRO, Lord Mayor's Waiting Book, 2, 29 March 1666; Clarendon, *Selections*, pp. 412–13.

110. R. Finlay, *Population and Metropolis. The Demography of London 1580–1650* (Cambridge, Cambridge University Press, 1981), p. 54.

111. Bell, *Great Plague*, pp. 150–1, 272; Champion, *London's Dreaded Visitation*, pp. 26–8.

112. This paragraph is based upon the data in Champion, *London's Dreaded Visitation*, pp. 27, 104–6; see also, Slack, *Impact of Plague*, pp. 154–64.

113. M.J. Power, 'The East and West in Early-Modern London', in E.W. Ives, R.J. Knecht and J.J. Scarisbrick (eds), *Wealth and Power in Tudor England* (London, Athlone Press, 1978), pp. 180–2.

114. M.J. Power, 'The social topography of Restoration London', in Beier and Finlay (eds), *London 1500–1700*, pp. 199–223.

115. Clarendon, *Selections*, p. 413; B. Capp, *Astrology and the Popular Press: English Almanacs 1500–1800* (London, Faber & Faber, 1979), p. 135.

116. Plummer, *London Weavers' Company*, p. 188.

117. Bell, *Great Plague*, p. 215; M. Duffy, *Henry Purcell* (London, Fourth Estate, 1994), p. 27.

118. I owe the information on Colt to the kindness of Adam White; O.L. Dick (ed.), *Aubrey's Brief Lives* (Harmondsworth, Penguin, 1972), p. 324.

119. Champion, *London's Dreaded Visitation*, pp. 53–62; Chester (ed.), *Parish Registers of St. Thomas the Apostle*, pp. 127–38; R.W. Herlan, 'Aspects of Population History in the London Parish of St. Olave, Old Jewry, 1645–1667', *Guildhall Studies in London History*, 4 (1980), 137.

120. *Diary of Pepys*, vol. 6, p. 342; BL, Add. MS 10,117, ff. 139–74; Nicholson, *Historical Sources*, pp. 150–1.

121. HMC, *Sixteenth Report, appendix: Manuscripts of the Earl of Verulam* (London, HMSO, 1906), p. 59; Plummer, *London Weavers' Company*, p. 188.

3. The Plague in the Provinces

1. HMC, *Thirteenth Report, Appendix IV* (London, HMSO, 1892), pp. 346–7; A.W. Langford, 'The Plague in Herefordshire', *Transactions of the Woolhope Naturalists' Field Club*, 25 (1955–7), 152–3.

2. H. Stocks (ed.), *Records of the Borough of Leicester . . ., 1603–1688* (Cambridge, Cambridge University Press, 1923), pp. 496, 503–4.

3. Slack, *Impact of Plague*, pp. 224–5.

4. VCH, *Lincolnshire*, vol. 2 (London, 1906), p. 340.

5. P.E. Jones (ed.), *The Fire Court* (2 vols, London, Corporation of London, 1966–70), vol. 1, p. 159; HMC, *Tenth Report, Appendix IV, Manuscripts of Captain Stewart*, p. 111; CLRO, Misc. MS 118/4.

6. Nicholson, *Historical Sources*, p. 24; *The London Gazette*, 10–14 May 1666.

7. VCH, *Staffordshire*, vol. 17 (London, 1976), p. 220; Nicholson, *Historical Sources*, pp. 22, 24; Bodl., MS Tanner 45, f. 26.

8. Nicholson, *Historical Sources*, pp. 25, 150; Slack, *Impact of Plague*, pp. 269, 294.

9. *CSPD*, 1665–6, p. 17.

10. VCH, *Middlesex*, vol. 9 (London, 1989), pp. 8–9.

11. Shrewsbury, *History of Bubonic Plague*, pp. 481, 483–4; A.G.E. Jones, 'The Great Plague in Croydon', *Notes and Queries*, 201 (1956), 332–4.

12. *Diary of Pepys*, vol. 6, p. 161; Shrewsbury, *History of Bubonic Plague*, p. 481.

13. A. Macfarlane (ed.), *The Diary of Ralph Josselin 1616–1683* (British Academy, Records of Social and Economic History, new series, III, 1976), pp. 518–21, 527.

14. F.G. Emmison, *Catalogue of Essex Parish Records 1240–1894* (Chelmsford, Essex County Council, 1966), p. 234.

15. M.J. Dobson, *A Chronology of Epidemic Disease and Mortality in Southeast England, 1601–1800* (Historical Geography Research Series, no. 19, 1990), p. 58; Slack, *Impact of Plague*, pp. 106,

289, 367 n.69; R. Barker, 'The local study of plague', *The Local Historian*, 14 (1981), 332–40; Emmison, *Essex Parish Records*, p. 41.

16. PRO, PC2/58, p. 267; PC2/59, pp. 6–7; *CSPD*, 1664–5, p. 505; 1665–6, p. 57.

17. VCH, *Essex*, vol. 9 (London, 1994), pp. 67–8, 77–87, 97–9; Israel, *Dutch Republic*, p. 625.

18. *Diary of Josselin*, p. 519.

19. *Diary of Josselin*, p. 520; L.C. Sier, 'Experiences of the Great Fire of London, 1666', *Essex Review*, 51 (1942), 134.

20. C. Creighton, *A History of Epidemics in Britain* (2 vols, London, Cass, 1965, original edn 1891–4), vol. I, pp. 688–9; I.G. Doolittle, 'The Plague in Colchester, 1579–1666', *Transactions of the Essex Archaeological Society*, 4 (1972), 141–3; *Diary of Josselin*, p. 522.

21. Creighton, *History of Epidemics*, vol. I, p. 690.

22. *Diary of Josselin*, pp. 523–5; VCH, *Essex*, vol. 9, p. 68.

23. Creighton, *History of Epidemics*, vol. I, pp. 689–90; another total of Morant's figures gives 5,259 deaths, of which 4,371 were from plague, Doolittle, 'Plague in Colchester', p. 137; *Diary of Pepys*, vol. 7, p. 193.

24. Manley, 'Central England temperatures', pp. 393–4; Lamb, *Climate: Present, Past and Future*, vol. 2, pp. 571–2; D.J. Schove, 'Fire and Drought, 1600–1700', *Weather*, 21 (1966), 313–14.

25. *Diary of Josselin*, p. 521; Dobson, *Chronology of Epidemic Disease*, p. 57; Shrewsbury, *History of Bubonic Plague*, p. 503.

26. *CSPD*, 1664–5, p. 505; Nicholson, *Historical Sources*, p. 24; M. Reed, 'Economic structure and change in seventeenth-century Ipswich', in P. Clark (ed.), *Country towns in pre-industrial England* (Leicester, Leicester University Press, 1981), pp. 92–6; Shrewsbury, *History of Bubonic Plague*, pp. 503–5; *Diary of Josselin*, p. 521.

27. Slack, *Impact of Plague*, pp. 106–7, 177, 367 nn.72, 73; Dobson, *Contours of death*, pp. 194, 282, 411.

28. J. Gyford, *Witham 1500–1700, Making a Living* (Witham, privately published, 1996), pp. 7–8; A.G.E. Jones, 'Plagues in Suffolk in the Seventeenth Century', *Notes and Queries*, 198 (1953), 384–6 and 'The Great Plague in Yarmouth', *Notes and Queries*, 202 (1957), 109.

29. Slack, *Impact of Plague*, pp. 66, 133; Jones, 'Great Plague in Yarmouth', 108–12; PRO, PC2/58, p. 130; HMC, *Ninth Report, Appendix I* (London, HMSO, 1883), p. 321; P. Gauci, *Politics and Society in Great Yarmouth 1660–1722* (Oxford, Oxford University Press, 1996), p. 27.

30. P. Corfield, 'A provincial capital in the late seventeenth century: The case of Norwich', in P. Clark and P. Slack (eds), *Crisis and Order in English Towns 1500–1700* (London, Routledge, 1972), pp. 263–310; *Diary of Evelyn*, p. 562.

31. Slack, *Impact of Plague*, pp. 126–37; U. Priestley, 'The Norwich Textile Industry: The London Connection', *The London Journal*, 19 (1994), 108–18.

32. *CSPD*, 1665–6, pp. 47, 252, 281.

33. R.H. Hill (ed.), *The Correspondence of Thomas Corie Town Clerk of Norwich, 1664–1687* (Norfolk Record Soc., vol. 27, 1956), p. 18.

34. *CSPD*, 1665–6, pp. 513, 568; 1666–7, pp. 2, 16, 53; *Correspondence of Thomas Corie*, pp. 18–19.

35. *CSPD*, 1666–7, pp. 393–4, 560, 564–5, 575; *Correspondence of Thomas Corie*, pp. 19–23.

36. *CSPD*, 1666–7, pp. 188, 393–4.

37. Slack, *Impact of Plague*, pp. 137–9.

38. Shrewsbury, *History of Bubonic Plague*, pp. 505, 513–14; VCH, *Cambridgeshire and the Isle of Ely*, vol. 4 (London, 1953), p. 44; Bedfordshire RO, Russell collection, box 291, G12/5, p. 3; PRO, E179/249/1; *Calendar of Treasury Books*, 1660–7, p. 732.

39. Shrewsbury, *History of Bubonic Plague*, p. 517; PRO, E179/254/11.

40. VCH, *Cambridgeshire and the Isle of Ely*, vol. 3 (London, 1959), p. 102; N. Goose, 'Household size and structure in early-Stuart Cambridge', in J. Barry (ed.), *The Tudor and Stuart Town: A Reader in English Urban History 1530–1688* (London, Longman, 1990), p. 81.

41. J.R. Wardale (ed.), *Clare College Letters and Documents* (Cambridge, Macmillan & Bowes, 1903), pp. 69–71; J.E. Foster (ed.), *The Diary of Samuel Newton Alderman of Cambridge (1662–1717)* (Cambridge Antiquarian Society, vol. 23, 1890), p. 16.

42. Shrewsbury, *History of Bubonic Plague*, p. 489; *Diary of Pepys*, vol. 6, pp. 195, 206; I. Roy, 'Greenwich and the Civil War', *Transactions of the Greenwich and Lewisham Antiquarian Society*, 10 (1985), 13.

43. *Diary of Evelyn*, p. 479; G. de la Bédoyère (ed.), *Particular Friends: The Correspondence of Samuel Pepys and John Evelyn* (Woodbridge, Boydell Press, 1997), pp. 36 n.4, 310; PRO, PC2/59, p. 108; Dobson, *Chronology of Epidemic Disease*, p. 56; BL, Add. MS 10,117, f. 174v.

44. Dobson, *Contours of death*, pp. 408–9; Shrewsbury, *History of Bubonic Plague*, pp. 488–92; PRO, PC2/59, pp. 118, 120, 519;.R. Marsh, *Rochester: The Evolution of the City and its Government* (Rochester, Medway Borough Council, 1976), pp. 37, 44; *Diary of Pepys*, vol. 7, p. 241; *CSPD*, 1665–6, p. 47.

45. Dobson, *Chronology of Epidemic Disease*, pp. 9, 59; 'Population, 1640–1831', in A. Armstrong (ed.), *The Economy of Kent, 1640–1914* (Woodbridge, Boydell Press and Kent County Council, 1995), pp. 21–3.

46. J. Taylor, 'Plague in the towns of Hampshire: the Epidemic of 1665–6', *Southern History*, 6 (1984), 104–12, 119–20.

47. PRO, PC2/58, pp. 209–10; BL, Add. MS 10,117, f. 145v; Taylor, 'Plague in the towns of Hampshire', 105–6, 109–14; A.T. Patterson, *A History of Southampton 1700–1914* (Southampton, Southampton University Press, 1966), pp. 2, 6.

48. *CSPD*, 1664–5, p. 504; M.J. Hoad (ed.), *Borough Sessions Papers 1653–1688* (Portsmouth Record Series, I, 1971), pp. 36, 41.

49. Taylor, 'Plague in the towns of Hampshire', pp. 109–17; *Diary of Pepys*, vol. 7, p. 41; Slack, *Impact of Plague*, p. 302; F.P. and M.M. Verney, *Memoirs of the Verney Family during the Seventeenth Century* (2nd edn, 2 vols, London, Longmans, Green, 1907), vol. 2, pp. 253–4.

50. Taylor, 'Plague in the towns of Hampshire', pp. 110, 114–15; A. Rosen, 'Winchester in transition, 1580–1700', in Clark (ed.), *Country towns* pp. 170–1; Shrewsbury, *History of Bubonic Plague*, p. 495.

51. *CSPD*, 1664–5, p. 499.

52. Shrewsbury, *History of Bubonic Plague*, pp. 496–8; Slack, *Impact of Plague*, p. 195; HMC, *Fifteenth Report, Report on Various Collections*, Volume I (London, HMSO, 1901), p. 148.

53. *CSPD*, 1665–6, p. 47; VCH, *Wiltshire*, vol. 5 (London, 1957), p. 320; Shrewsbury, *History of Bubonic Plague*, p. 498; HMC, *Fifteenth Report, Various Collections*, pp. 147–8.

54. Slack, *Impact of Plague*, p. 318; Bell, *Great Plague*, p. 322; PRO, PC2/59, p. 70.

55. Shrewsbury, *History of Bubonic Plague*, p. 499; N.C. Oswald, 'Epidemics in Devon, 1538–1837', *Transactions of the Devonshire Association*, 109 (1977), 95; Slack, *Impact of Plague*, pp. 317, 420 n.14.

56. HMC, *Seventeenth Report: Finch Manuscripts, I* (London, HMSO, 1913), p. 433.

57. Shrewsbury, *History of Bubonic Plague*, p. 530.

58. Langford, 'Plague in Herefordshire', 153; L.G. Schwoerer, *Lady Rachel Russell 'One of the Best of Women'* (Baltimore, John Hopkins University Press, 1988), pp. 20, 29.

59. I owe this information to the kindness of Gordon Forster.

60. Slack, *Impact of Plague*, p. 395 n.108; Bodl., Add. MS c.303, ff. 122, 124; Bell, *Great Plague*, pp. 300–1; PRO, PC 2/58, p. 257; *CSPD*, 1665–6, p. 53; HMC, *Manuscripts of the Marquess of Bath* (London, HMSO, 1968), p. 255.

61. BL, Add. MS 11,042, f. 115; HMC, *Fourteenth Report, Part II: Portland Manuscripts, III* (London, HMSO, 1894), p. 293.

62. HMC, *Fifteenth Report, appendix: Manuscripts of J.M. Heathcote* (London, HMSO, 1899), p. 216.

63. VCH, *Berkshire*, vol. 3 (London, 1923), pp. 62, 362; *Calendar of Treasury Books*, 1660–7, p. 732; Shrewsbury, *History of Bubonic Plague*, p. 518.

64. Shrewsbury, *History of Bubonic Plague*, p. 481; VCH, *Buckinghamshire*, vol. 3 (London, 1925), p. 114.

65. J.A. Dils, 'Epidemics, Mortality, and the Civil War in Berkshire, 1642–6', in R.C. Richardson (ed.), *The English Civil Wars, Local Aspects* (Stroud, Sutton, 1997), p. 148.

66. VCH, *Buckinghamshire*, vol. 4 (London, 1927), p. 276; Shrewsbury, *History of Bubonic Plague*, p. 518.

67. S. Bond, 'The Plague at Northampton', *Northamptonshire Past and Present*, 3 (1965–6), 276–7; Wilshere, 'Plague in Leicester', p. 64; K.R. Adey, 'Seventeenth-century Stafford: A County Town in Decline', *Midland History*, 2 (1974), 162–3; Slack, *Impact of Plague*, p. 303.

68. William Hutton, *The History of Birmingham* (Birmingham, 1835), p. 29 and *The History of Derby* (2nd edn, London, 1817), pp. 194–5; Shrewsbury, *History of Bubonic Plague*, pp. 518–22; L. Bradley, 'The Most Famous Of All English Plagues: A detailed analysis of the Plague at Eyam, 1665–6', in *The Plague Reconsidered*, p. 69.

69. Shrewsbury, *History of Bubonic Plague*, p. 536.

70. *Calendar of Treasury Books*, 1660–7, p. 731.

71. Wilshere, 'Plague in Leicester', pp. 63–4.

72. Bradley, 'The Most Famous Of All English Plagues', pp. 64–5, 68–9, 80; P. Race, 'Some further consideration of the Plague in Eyam 1665/6', *Local Population Studies*, 54 (1995), 57.

73. J.G. and F. Clifford (eds), *Eyam Parish Register 1630–1700* (Derbyshire Record Soc., 21, 1993), pp. vii, 87–98; Bradley, 'The Most Famous Of All English Plagues', pp. 67–8, 70–2, 76–7, 80; Race, 'Plague in Eyam', 58–9.

74. Bradley, 'The Most Famous Of All English Plagues', pp. 72–5, 91–3.

75. G. Ornsby (ed.), *The Correspondence of John Cosin, D.D. Lord Bishop of Durham*, pt II (Surtees Society, LV, 1872), pp. 134, 138.

76.   *Correspondence of John Cosin*, pp. 134, 143, 161–2, 167; Nicholson, *Historical Sources*, pp. 139, 150–1; HMC, *Twelfth Report, Manuscripts of S.H. Le Fleming* (London, HMSO, 1890), pp. 37–8; Dobson, 'Population, 1640–1831', p. 22.

4. Policy and Plague

1.   *CSPD*, 1655, pp. 322–3.
2.   PRO, PC2/56, p. 592; *CSPD*, 1664–5, pp. 150–1.
3.   PRO, PC2/56, pp. 610, 612.
4.   PRO, PC2/56, pp. 676, 683, 688 and PC2/57, pp. 89, 93, 126–8, 164, 199–200, 305.
5.   *CSPD*, 1655, p. 381; PRO, PC 2/57, pp. 104, 126, 186.
6.   PRO, PC2/57, pp. 23, 45, 132, 139, 177, 218–19, 220, 235, 237, 245, 278–9.
7.   *CSPD*, 1664–5, p. 287; PRO, PC2/57, pp. 261, 306, 328; J.R. Jones, *The Anglo-Dutch Wars of the Seventeenth Century* (London, Longman, 1996), p. 151.
8.   PRO, PC2/58, pp. 114, 135, 141–3.
9.   LMA, WC/R/1, pp. 2–7.
10.   LMA, WC/R/1, pp. 2, 4–6.
11.   Bell, *Great Plague*, pp. 26–7, 131.
12.   Bodl., Add. MS c.303, f. 112; Slack, *Impact of Plague*, pp. 297–8.
13.   *CSPD*, 1664–5, pp. 504, 506–7; PRO, PC2/58, p. 188; Bell, *Great Plague*, pp. 194–5, 324.
14.   J.C. Jeaffreson (ed.), *Middlesex County Records*, III (London, Middlesex County Records Society, 1888), p. 375.
15.   P. Slack, 'Books of Orders: the Making of English Social Policy, 1577–1631', *Transactions of the Royal Historical Society*, 5th series, 30 (1980), 18; G.C.F. Forster, 'Government in Provincial England under the Later Stuarts', *Transactions of the Royal Historical Society*, 5th series, 33 (1983), 35.
16.   Nicholson, *Historical Sources*, p. 130; CLRO, Lord Mayor's Waiting Book, 2, 22 September 1665.
17.   Nicholson, *Historical Sources*, pp. 131, 134; *CSPD*, 1664–5, p. 401.
18.   Nicholson, *Historical Sources*, pp. 132, 134–5.
19.   Nicholson, *Historical Sources*, pp. 104, 106; Slack, *Impact of Plague*, pp. 250–1.
20.   PRO, SP29/126/44.
21.   Hull (ed.), *Economic Writings* vol. 1, pp. 108–10.
22.   Pullan, 'Plague and perceptions of the poor', pp. 120–1.
23.   Bell, *Great Plague*, pp. 315–16.
24.   Jeaffreson (ed.), *Middlesex County Records*, III, pp. 373–5.
25.   PRO, PC2/58, p. 347; *CSPD*, 1665–6, p. 351.
26.   F.H.W. Sheppard (ed.), *Survey of London, Vol. 31, The Parish of St James, Westminster* (London, Athlone, 1963), p. 196.
27.   Bell, *Great Plague*, pp. 315–18; Slack, 'Metropolitan government in crisis', p. 67.
28.   Bell, *Great Plague*, pp. 315–18; Slack, 'Metropolitan government in crisis', p. 73; Jeaffreson (ed.), *Middlesex County Records*, III, pp. 372–3, 375, 377, 379; PRO, PC2/58, pp. 118, 345–7, 390–1.

29. Bell, *Great Plague*, pp. 333–5; PRO, PC2/59, p. 13.

30. Bell, *Great Plague*, pp. 334–5; Jeaffreson (ed.), *Middlesex County Records*, III, pp. 373–4.

31. D. Pickering (ed.), *The Statutes at Large*, VII (London, 1763), pp. 141–4.

32. *Commons' Journals*, VIII, 1660–7, pp. 614, 623–4, 641, 663–4, 687; *Lords' Journals*, XI, 1660–6, pp. 689, 698; *Lords' Journals*, XII, 1666–75, pp. 86, 102.

33. Hutton, *The Restoration*, pp. 233–6; J. Miller, *Charles II* (London, Weidenfeld & Nicolson, 1991), pp. 110–11, 120.

34. Clarendon, *Selections*, p. 455.

35. *CSPD*, 1664–5, p. 473 and 1665–6, p. 111; P. Hume Brown (ed.), *The Register of the Privy Council of Scotland, third series, II, 1665–1669* (Edinburgh, HMSO, 1909), pp. 71–4, 95, 147–8; C.F. Mullett, 'Plague Policy in Scotland, 16th-17th Centuries', *Osiris*, 9 (1950), pp. 452–3.

36. HMC, *Seventeenth Report, Appendix, Diocese of Gloucester* (London, HMSO, 1914), p. 64; R.V. Lennard, 'English Agriculture under Charles II', in W.E. Minchinton (ed.), *Essays in Agrarian History*, Vol. 1, (Newton Abbot, David & Charles, 1968), p. 167; LMA, acc.262/43/47; *CSPD*, 1665–6, pp. 14, 17.

37. Bell, *Great Plague*, p. 187; Taylor, 'Plague in the towns of Hampshire', 114.

38. Bell, *Great Plague*, p. 188.

39. *CSPD*, 1664–5, p. 571 and 1665–6, pp. 56–7; C.D. Chandaman, *The English Public Revenue 1660–1688* (Oxford, Oxford University Press, 1975), p. 15 n.1.

40. *CSPD*, 1665–6, pp. 56–7; *The London Gazette*, 26–30 April and 3–7 May 1666; PRO, PC2/59, p. 70.

41. PRO, PC2/58, p. 394; *CSPD*, 1664–5, p. 488.

42. *CSPD*, 1664–5, p. 571 and 1665–6, p. 107.

43. *Correspondence of John Cosin*, pp. 151, 164.

44. LMA, acc.262/43/51, 63.

45. *Correspondence of Thomas Corie*, p. 19; *Correspondence of John Cosin*, p. 151; HMC, *Fifteenth Report, Various Collections*, I, p. 148.

46. I.G. Doolittle, 'The effects of the plague on a provincial town in the sixteenth and seventeenth centuries', *Medical History*, 19 (1975), 335; Reed, 'Seventeenth-century Ipswich', pp. 123, 135.

47. PRO, PC2/59, pp. 6–7.

48. *Diary of Pepys*, vol. 6, pp. 165, 168, 186, 192, 205, 207, 224, 233, 268, 278, 293; Howarth (ed.), *Letters and Second Diary of Samuel Pepys*, pp. 24–5; A. Saunders (ed.), *The Royal Exchange* (London Topographical Society, 152, 1997), pp. 87, 198–202.

49. Jones, *Anglo-Dutch Wars*, p. 57.

50. *Diary of Pepys*, vol. 6, pp. 266–7.

51. Chandaman, *English Public Revenue*, pp. 89–91, 318–19.

52. Chandaman, *English Public Revenue*, pp. 23, 55–7, 132, 179–80, 211, 223, 312; *Calendar of Treasury Books*, 1660–7, p. 710; Taylor, 'Plague in the towns of Hampshire', 115.

53. *Diary of Pepys*, vol. 6, p. 255.

54. *Diary of Pepys*, vol. 6, p. 218; de la Bédoyère (ed.), *Particular Friends*, p. 36 n.4.

55. Jones, *Anglo-Dutch Wars*, pp. 57–60.

56.   Jones, *Anglo-Dutch Wars*, pp. 166–78; S. Porter, *The Great Fire of London* (Stroud, Sutton, 1996), pp. 69–74, 90–1.

57.   Chandaman, *English Public Revenue*, pp. 210–13.

5. The Great Plague in Perspective

1.   G.E. Christianson, *In the Presence of the Creator: Isaac Newton and His Times* (New York, The Free Press, 1984), pp. 68, 72–4.

2.   J.A. Winn, *John Dryden and His World* (New Haven and London, Yale University Press, 1987), pp. 157–9; *Aubrey's Brief Lives*, p. 382.

3.   Race, 'Plague in Eyam', pp. 60–2.

4.   Shrewsbury, *History of Bubonic Plague*, p. 478.

5.   Porter, *Great Fire*, pp. 111–12, 127.

6.   Hull (ed.), *Economic Writings*, vol. 2, pp. 367, 376.

7.   VCH, *Essex*, vol. 9, pp. 67–8, 77, 81–7; Dobson, *Contours of Death*, p. 485.

8.   Reed, 'Seventeenth-century Ipswich', pp. 94–5, 102–5, 125; Morris (ed.), *Journeys of Celia Fiennes*, p. 132.

9.   Morris (ed.), *Journeys of Celia Fiennes*, p. 137; Corfield, 'A provincial capital', pp. 266–72, 286.

10.   Morris (ed.), *Journeys of Celia Fiennes*, pp. 73, 123; M. Exwood and H.L. Lehmann (eds), *The Journal of William Schellinks' Travels in England 1661–1663* (Camden Society, 5th series, I, 1993), p. 138; Patterson, *History of Southampton*, pp. 2–6.

11.   Rosen, 'Winchester in transition', pp. 170–1; Daniel Defoe, *A Tour through the Whole Island of Great Britain*, ed. P. Rogers (Harmondsworth, Penguin, 1971), pp. 191–2.

12.   J. Thirsk (ed.), *The Agrarian History of England and Wales, Volume V, 1640–1750: II. Agrarian Change* (Cambridge, Cambridge University Press, 1985), p. 76.

13.   J. Patten, 'Patterns of migration and movement of labour to three pre-industrial East Anglian towns', *Journal of Historical Geography*, 2 (1976), 118–28.

14.   Thirsk (ed.), *Agrarian History*, pp. 828–9, 847.

15.   E.A. Wrigley and R.S. Schofield, *The Population History of England 1541–1871* (London, Arnold, 1981) pp. 208–9.

16.   E.A. Wrigley, 'A simple model of London's importance in changing English society and economy 1650–1750', *Past and Present*, 37 (1967), 47–9; Hull (ed.), *Economic Writings*, vol. 2, pp. 376–7.

17.   S. Porter, 'University and Society', in N. Tyacke (ed.), *The History of the University of Oxford, Volume IV, Seventeenth-Century Oxford* (Oxford, Clarendon Press, 1997), p. 46; Hull (ed.), *Economic Writings*, vol. 2, pp. 475–6.

18.   D.V. Glass, *Numbering the people* (Farnborough, Heath, 1973), p. 37 n.76.

19.   Wrigley and Schofield, *Population History of England*, pp. 333, 653, 674–5.

20.   Dobson, *Contours of death*, p. 380.

21.   Sutherland, 'When was the Great Plague?', pp. 287–313.

22.   Sprat, *History of the Royal Society*, p. 123.

23.   Slack, *Impact of Plague*, pp. 248–9.

24.   Mullett, *Bubonic Plague and England*, pp. 259–61.

25. Mullett, *Bubonic Plague and England*, p. 262; *Aubrey's Brief Lives*, pp. 210–11.

26. J. Meuvret, 'Demographic Crisis in France from the Sixteenth to the Eighteenth Century', in D.V. Glass and D.E.C. Eversley (eds), *Population in History* (London, Arnold, 1965), p. 515; Roseveare (ed.), *Markets and Merchants*, p. 88.

27. J. Stoye, *Europe Unfolding, 1648–1688* (London, Collins, 1969), p. 319; *Marsigli's Europe 1680–1730. The Life and Times of Luigi Ferdinando Marsigli, Soldier and Virtuoso* (New Haven and London, Yale University Press, 1994), p. 19.

28. H. Kamen, *Spain 1469–1714: A society in conflict* (London, Longman, 1991), p. 270; Slack, *Impact of Plague*, p. 324.

29. D. Kirby, *Northern Europe in the Early Modern Period: The Baltic World 1492–1772* (London, Longman, 1990), p. 352; Mullett, *Bubonic Plague and England*, p. 264.

30. Jonathan Swift, *Journal to Stella*, ed. H. Williams (2 vols, Oxford, Clarendon Press, 1948), vol. 1, pp. 115–16, 118 and vol. 2, p. 564; Slack, *Impact of Plague*, p. 324; Sheppard (ed.), *The Survey of London*, vol. 31, p. 196.

31. R. West, *The Life & Strange Surprising Adventures of Daniel Defoe* (London, HarperCollins, 1997), pp. 266–70.

32. PRO, PC2/86, pp. 472, 475, 476–80; PC2/87, pp. 15–17, 27–35, 122–31, 313–17.

33. Stoye, *Marsigli's Europe*, p. 292; PRO, PC2/87, *passim*.

34. PRO, PC2/87, pp. 323–4, 327, 341–3, 351.

35. Slack, *Impact of Plague*, pp. 327–8, 333–4; PRO, PC2/87, pp. 321, 327.

36. PRO, PC2/87, pp. 324, 341, 343, 451.

37. Slack, *Impact of Plague*, pp. 328–33; Pickering (ed.), *Statutes at Large*, vol. 14, pp. 302–3, 380–3.

38. Pickering (ed.), *Statutes at Large*, vol. 21, pp. 15, 53.

39. A. Corbin, *The Foul and the Fragrant: Odour and the Social Imagination* (London, Macmillan, 1996), pp. 62–3, 66, 211–12, 252 n.76.

40. McNeill, *Plagues and Peoples*, p. 216.

41. P. Mansel, *Constantinople, City of the World's Desire 1453–1924* (London, John Murray, 1995), pp. 225–6, 256.

42. Daniel Defoe, *Memoirs of a Cavalier*, ed. J.T. Boulton (Oxford, Oxford University Press, 1991), pp. 28–9.

43. P.R. Backscheider, *Daniel Defoe His Life* (Baltimore and London, John Hopkins University Press, 1989), p. 489.

44. Slack, *Impact of Plague*, p. 335; W. Besant, *London in the Time of the Stuarts* (London, Adams & Black, 1903), pp. 223–4; Daniel Defoe, *A Journal of the Plague Year*, ed. A. Burgess (Harmondsworth, Penguin, 1966), pp. 14–15.

45. Nicholson, *Historical Sources*, p. 100.

46. Howarth (ed.), *Letters and Second Diary of Samuel Pepys*, p. 25.

47. D. Esterly, *Grinling Gibbons and the Art of Carving* (London, V&A Publications, 1998), p. 12.

48. Defoe, *Tour*, pp. 58–9; Doolittle, 'Plague in Colchester', 137–8.

49. Bradley, 'The Most Famous Of All English Plagues', pp. 63–4, 80.

50. Maddicott, 'Plague in seventh-century England', p. 45.

51. W. Besant, *London in the Time of the Stuarts* (London, Adams & Black, 1903), p. 233.

52. Wills, *Plagues*, p. 70.

53. S. Schama, *The Embarrassment of Riches. An Interpretation of Dutch Culture in the Golden Age* (London, Collins, 1987), pp. 377–8.

54. G. Karlsson, 'Plague without rats: the case of fifteenth-century Iceland', *Journal of Medieval History*, 22 (1996), 276–7.

55. Lamb, *Climate*, vol. 2, pp. 572–3; G. Manley, '1684: The Coldest Winter in the English Historical Record', *Weather*, 30 (1975), 382–8.

56. Robert Southey, *Letters from England*, ed. J. Simmons (Gloucester, Sutton, 1984), pp. 138–9; A.B. Appleby, 'The Disappearance of Plague: A continuing Puzzle', *Economic History Review*, 33 (1980), 167.

57. Appleby, 'Disappearance of Plague', pp. 169–73; P. Slack, 'The Disappearance of Plague: An Alternative View', *Economic History Review*, 34 (1981), 470.

58. Appleby, 'Disappearance of Plague', 164; Champion, *London's Dreaded Visitation*, pp. 81–2, 98–9; Cabbages and Kings: The Great Dog Massacre, BBC Radio 4, 26 April 1997.

59. Slack, 'Disappearance of Plague', p. 474.

60. Slack, *Impact of Plague*, p. 421 n.34.

61. McNeill, *Plagues and Peoples*, p. 141.

62. Shrewsbury, *History of Bubonic Plague*, pp. 506–10, 531–2, 535–6.

63. *The Annual Register*, vol. 9 (1766), p. 104.

Bibliography

Adey, K.R., 'Seventeenth-century Stafford: A County Town in Decline', *Midland History*, 2 (1974), 152–67

Appleby, A.B. , 'The Disappearance of Plague: A continuing Puzzle', *Economic History Review*, 33 (1980), 161–73

Aubrey: *Aubrey's Brief Lives*, ed. O.L. Dick, Harmondsworth, Penguin, 1972

Backscheider, P.R., *Daniel Defoe His Life*, Baltimore and London, John Hopkins University Press, 1989

Ballon, H., *The Paris of Henri IV: Architecture and Urbanism*, Cambridge, Mass., MIT Press, 1991

Barker, R., 'The local study of plague', *The Local Historian*, 14 (1981), 332–40

Baxter, *Calendar of the Correspondence of Richard Baxter, Volume II 1660–1696*, eds N.H. Keble and G.F. Nuttall, Oxford, Oxford University Press, 1991

Bédoyère, G. de la (ed.), *The Writings of John Evelyn*, Woodbridge, Boydell Press, 1995

—— (ed.), *Particular Friends: The Correspondence of Samuel Pepys and John Evelyn*, Woodbridge, Boydell Press, 1997

Beier, A.L. and Finlay, R. (eds), *London 1500–1700: The making of the metropolis*, London, Longman, 1986

Bell, John, *London's Remembrancer: or, A true Accompt of every particular Weeks Christnings and Mortality In all the Years of Pestilence . . .* , (1665)

Bell, W.G., *The Great Plague in London*, London, Bodley Head, 1924, reprinted London, Bracken Books, 1994

Besant, W., *London in the Time of the Stuarts*, London, Adams & Black, 1903

Biraben, J.N., 'Current Medical and Epidemiological Views on Plague', in Local Population Studies, *The Plague Reconsidered*

Bond, S., 'The Plague at Northampton', *Northamptonshire Past and Present*, 3 (1965–6), 276–7

Borsay, P., *The English Urban Renaissance: Culture and Society in the Provincial Town, 1660–1770*, Oxford, Clarendon Press, 1989

Bradley, L., 'The Most Famous Of All English Plagues: A detailed analysis of the Plague at Eyam, 1665–6', in Local Population Studies, *The Plague Reconsidered*

Brown, J.C., *In the Shadow of Florence: Provincial Society in Renaissance Pescia*, Oxford, Oxford University Press, 1982

Burnby, J.G.L., *A Study of the English Apothecary from 1660 to 1760*, London, *Medical History*, supplement no. 3, 1983

Burnet, Gilbert, *History of His Own Time*, London, Dent, 1991

Capp, B., *Astrology and the Popular Press: English Almanacs 1500–1800*, London, Faber & Faber, 1979

Carlton, C., *Going to the Wars. The Experience of the British Civil Wars, 1638–1651*, London, Routledge, 1992

Champion, J.A.I. (ed.), *Epidemic Disease in London*, London, Centre for Metropolitan History, Working Paper Series, no. 1, 1993

——, *London's Dreaded Visitation. The Social Geography of the Great Plague in 1665*, London, Historical Geography Research Series, 31, 1995

Chandaman, C.D., *The English Public Revenue 1660–1688*, Oxford, Oxford University Press, 1975

Chester, J.L. (ed.), *The Parish Registers of St. Thomas the Apostle, London . . . 1558 to 1754*, London, Harleian Society, parish registers, vol. VI, 1881

Christianson, G.E., *In the Presence of the Creator: Isaac Newton and His Times*, New York, The Free Press, 1984

Cipolla, C.M., 'The Plague and the Pre-Malthus Malthusians', *Journal of European Economic History*, 3 (1974), 277–84

——, *Public Health and the Medical Profession in the Renaissance*, Cambridge, Cambridge University Press, 1976

——, *Fighting the Plague in Seventeenth-Century Italy*, Madison, University of Wisconsin Press, 1981

Clarendon, Edward Hyde, Earl of Clarendon, *Selections from The History of the Rebellion and The Life by Himself*, ed. G. Huehns, Oxford, Oxford University Press, 1978

Clark, P. (ed.), *Country towns in pre-industrial England*, Leicester, Leicester University Press, 1981

—— and Slack, P. (eds), *Crisis and Order in English Towns 1500–1700*, London, Routledge, 1972

Clifford, J.G. and F. (eds), *Eyam Parish Register 1630–1700*, Derbyshire Record Society, 21, 1993

Cooper, W.D., 'Notices of the last Great Plague, 1665–6; from the Letters of John Allin to Philip Fryth and Samuel Jeake', *Archaeologia*, 37 (1857), 1–22

Corbin, A., *The Foul and the Fragrant: Odour and the Social Imagination*, London, Macmillan, 1996

Corfield, P., 'A provincial capital in the late seventeenth century: The case of Norwich', in P. Clark and P. Slack (eds), *Crisis and Order in English Towns 1500–1700*, London, Routledge, 1972

Creighton, C., *A History of Epidemics in Britain*, 2 vols, London, Cass, 1965, original edn 1891–4

Cunliffe, B., *The City of Bath*, Stroud, Sutton, 1986

Defoe, Daniel, *A Journal of the Plague Year*, ed. A. Burgess, Harmondsworth, Penguin, 1966

—— *A Tour through the Whole Island of Great Britain*, ed. P. Rogers, Harmondsworth, Penguin, 1971

—— *Memoirs of a Cavalier*, ed. J.T. Boulton, Oxford, Oxford University Press, 1991

Dils, J.A., 'Epidemics, Mortality, and the Civil War in Berkshire, 1642–6', in R.C. Richardson (ed.), *The English Civil Wars, Local Aspects*, Stroud, Sutton, 1997

Dobson, M.J., *A Chronology of Epidemic Disease and Mortality in Southeast England, 1601–1800*, Historical Geography Research Series, no. 19, 1990

—— 'Population, 1640–1831', in A. Armstrong (ed.), *The Economy of Kent, 1640–1914*, Woodbridge, Boydell Press and Kent County Council, 1995

—— *Contours of death and disease in early modern England*, Cambridge, Cambridge University Press, 1997

Doolittle, I.G., 'The Plague in Colchester, 1579–1666', *Transactions of the Essex Archaeological Society*, 4 (1972), 134–45

—— 'The effects of the plague on a provincial town in the sixteenth and seventeenth centuries', *Medical History*, 19 (1975), 333–41

Duffy, M., *Henry Purcell*, London, Fourth Estate, 1994

Duplessis, R.S., *Lille and the Dutch revolt: Urban Stability in an Era of Revolution 1500–1582*, Cambridge, Cambridge University Press, 1991

Dyer, A.D., *The City of Worcester in the sixteenth century*, Leicester, Leicester University Press, 1973

Emmison, F.G., *Catalogue of Essex Parish Records 1240–1894*, Chelmsford, Essex County Council, 1966

Esterly, D., *Grinling Gibbons and the Art of Carving*, London, V&A Publications, 1998

Evelyn, *The Diary of John Evelyn*, ed. E.S. de Beer, London, Oxford University Press, 1959

Exwood, M. and Lehmann, H.L. (eds), *The Journal of William Schellinks' Travels in England 1661–1663*, Camden Society, 5th series, I, 1993

Fiennes, *The Illustrated Journeys of Celia Fiennes 1685–c. 1712*, ed. C. Morris, Stroud, Alan Sutton Publishing, 1995

Finlay, R., *Population and Metropolis. The Demography of London 1580–1650*, Cambridge, Cambridge University Press, 1981

—— and Shearer, B., 'Population growth and suburban expansion' in A.L. Beier and R. Finlay (eds), *London 1500–1700: The making of the metropolis*

Forster, G.C.F., 'Government in Provincial England under the Later Stuarts', *Transactions of the Royal Historical Society*, 5th series, 33 (1983), 29–48

Foster, J.E. (ed.), *The Diary of Samuel Newton Alderman of Cambridge (1662–1717)*, Cambridge Antiquarian Society, vol. 23, 1890

Frith, B., 'Some aspects of the history of medicine in Gloucestershire, 1500–1800', *Transactions of the Bristol and Gloucestershire Archaeological Society*, 108 (1990), 5–16

Gardiner, D. (ed.), *The Oxinden and Peyton Letters 1642–1670*, London, Sheldon Press, 1937

Gauci, P., *Politics and Society in Great Yarmouth 1660–1722*, Oxford, Oxford University Press, 1996

Gillett, E. and MacMahon, K.A., *A History of Hull*, Hull, Hull University Press, 1985

Gittings, C., *Death, Burial and the Individual in Early Modern England*, London, Routledge, 1984

Glass, D.V., *Numbering the people*, Farnborough, Heath, 1973

Godfrey, W.H., *The Church of Saint Bride, Fleet Street*, London, Survey of London, Monograph No. 15, 1944

Goose, N., 'Household size and structure in early-Stuart Cambridge', in J. Barry (ed.), *The Tudor and Stuart Town: A Reader in English Urban History 1530–1688*, London, Longman, 1990

Gyford, J., *Witham 1500–1700, Making a Living*, Witham, privately published, 1996

Haks, D. and van der Sman, M.C. (eds), *Dutch Society in the Age of Vermeer*, Zwolle, Waanders, 1996

Harding, V., '"And one more may be laid there": the Location of Burials in Early Modern London', *The London Journal*, 14 (1989), 112–29

—— 'Burial of the plague dead in early modern London', in J.A.I. Champion (ed.), *Epidemic Disease in London*

—— 'The Population of London, 1550–1700: a review of the published evidence', *The London Journal*, 15 (1990), 111–28

Hatcher, J., *Plague, Population and the English Economy 1348–1530*, London, Macmillan, 1977, reprinted in M. Anderson (ed.), *British population history from the Black Death to the present day*, Cambridge, Cambridge University Press, 1996

Herlan, R.W., 'Aspects of Population History in the London Parish of St. Olave, Old Jewry, 1645–1667', *Guildhall Studies in London History*, 4 (1980), 133–40

Hill, R.W. (ed.), *The Correspondence of Thomas Corie Town Clerk of Norwich, 1664–1687*, Norfolk Record Society, vol. 27, 1956

HMC *Sixth Report, MSS of the Duke of Northumberland*, London, HMSO, 1877

—— *Ninth Report, Appendix I*, London, HMSO, 1883

—— *Tenth Report, Appendix IV, Manuscripts of Captain Stewart*, London, HMSO, 1885

—— *Twelfth Report, Manuscripts of S.H. Le Fleming*, London, HMSO, 1890

—— *Thirteenth Report, Appendix IV*, London, HMSO, 1892

—— *Fourteenth Report, Part II: Portland Manuscripts, III*, London, HMSO, 1894

—— *Fifteenth Report, appendix: Manuscripts of J.M. Heathcote*, London, HMSO, 1899

—— *Fifteenth Report, Report on Various Collections*, Volume I, London, HMSO, 1901

—— *Sixteenth Report, appendix: Manuscripts of the Earl of Verulam*, London, HMSO, 1906

—— *Seventeenth Report: Finch Manuscripts, I*, London, HMSO, 1913

—— *Seventeenth Report, Appendix, Diocese of Gloucester*, London, HMSO, 1914

—— *Manuscripts of the Marquess of Bath*, London, HMSO, 1968

Hoad, M.J. (ed.), *Borough Sessions Papers 1653–1688*, Portsmouth Record Series, I, 1971

Horrox, R. (ed.), *The Black Death*, Manchester, Manchester University Press, 1994

Howel, James, *Londinopolis*, London, 1658

Hutton, R., *The Restoration. A Political and Religious History of England and Wales 1658–1667*, Oxford, Oxford University Press, 1985

Hutton, William, *The History of Birmingham*, Birmingham, 1835

—— *The History of Derby*, 2nd edn, London, 1817

Israel, J., *The Dutch Republic: Its Rise, Greatness, and Fall, 1477–1806*, Oxford, Clarendon Press, 1995

Jeaffreson, J.C. (ed.), *Middlesex County Records*, III, London, Middlesex County Records Society, 1888

Jenner, M.S.R., 'The Great Dog Massacre', in W.G. Naphy and P. Roberts (eds), *Fear in early modern society*, Manchester, University of Manchester Press, 1997

Jones, A.G.E., 'Plagues in Suffolk in the Seventeenth Century', *Notes and Queries*, 198 (1953), 384–6

—— 'The Great Plague in Croydon', *Notes and Queries*, 201 (1956), 332–4

—— 'The Great Plague in Yarmouth', *Notes and Queries*, 202 (1957), 108–12

Jones, P.E. (ed.), *The Fire Court*, 2 vols, London, Corporation of London, 1966–70

Jones, J.R., *The Anglo-Dutch Wars of the Seventeenth Century*, London, Longman, 1996

Josselin, *The Diary of Ralph Josselin 1616–1683*, ed. A. Macfarlane, British Academy, Records of Social and Economic History, new series, III, 1976

Kamen, H., *Spain 1469–1714: A society in conflict*, London, Longman, 1991

Karlsson, G., 'Plague without rats: the case of fifteenth-century Iceland', *Journal of Medieval History*, 22 (1996), 263–84

Kirby, D., *Northern Europe in the Early Modern Period: The Baltic World 1492–1772*, London, Longman, 1990

Ladurie, E. Le Roy, *The Peasants of Languedoc*, Urbana, University of Illinois Press, 1976

Lamb, H.H., *Climate: Present, Past and Future*, 2 vols, London, Methuen, 1972–7

Langford, A.W., 'The Plague in Herefordshire', *Transactions of the Woolhope Naturalists' Field Club*, 25 (1955–7), 146–53

Larkin, J.F. (ed.), *Stuart Royal Proclamations Volume II: Royal Proclamations of King Charles I 1625–1646*, Oxford, Oxford University Press, 1983

—— and Hughes, P.L. (eds), *Stuart Royal Proclamations Volume I: Royal Proclamations of King James I 1603–1625*, Oxford, Oxford University Press, 1973

Lennard, R.V., 'English Agriculture under Charles II', in W.E. Minchinton (ed.), *Essays in Agrarian History*, Vol. 1, Newton Abbot, David & Charles, 1968

Local Population Studies, *The Plague Reconsidered: A new look at its origins and effects in 16th and 17th Century England*, Matlock, Local Population Studies Supplement, 1977

Longstaffe, W.H.D. (ed.), *Memoirs of the Life of Mr. Ambrose Barnes*, Surtees Society, vol. 50, 1867

Maddicot, J.R., 'Plague in Seventh-Century England', *Past and Present*, 156 (1997), 9–54

Manley, G., 'Central England temperatures: monthly means 1659 to 1973', *Quarterly Journal of the Royal Meteorological Society*, 100 (1974), 389–405

—— '1684: The Coldest Winter in the English Historical Record', *Weather*, 30 (1975), 382–8

Mansel, P., *Constantinople, City of the World's Desire 1453–1924*, London, John Murray, 1995

Marsh, R., *Rochester: The Evolution of the City and its Government*, Rochester, Medway Borough Council, 1976

McNeill, W.H., *Plagues and Peoples*, New York, Doubleday, 1989

Meuvret, J., 'Demographic Crisis in France from the Sixteenth to the Eighteenth Century' in D.V. Glass and D.E.C. Eversley (eds), *Population in History* London, Arnold, 1965

Miller, J., *Charles II*, London, Weidenfeld & Nicolson, 1991

Morris, C., 'The Plague', in R.C. Latham and W. Matthews (eds), *The Diary of Samuel Pepys*, vol. 10

Mullett, C.F., 'Plague Policy in Scotland, 16th–17th Centuries', *Osiris*, 9 (1950), 435–56

—— *The Bubonic Plague and England*, Lexington, University of Kentucky Press, 1956

Nicholson, W., *The Historical Sources of Defoe's Journal of the Plague Year*, Boston, Mass., Stratford, 1919

Oldenburg, *The Correspondence of Henry Oldenburg*, A.R. and M.B. Hall (eds), 13 vols, Madison, University of Wisconsin Press, 1965–86

Ornsby, G. (ed.), *The Correspondence of John Cosin, D.D. Lord Bishop of Durham*, pt II, Surtees Society, LV, 1872

Oswald, N.C., 'Epidemics in Devon, 1538–1837', *Transactions of the Devonshire Association*, 109 (1977), 73–116

Parker, G., *The Army of Flanders and the Spanish Road 1567–1659*, Cambridge, Cambridge University Press, 1972

—— *Europe in Crisis, 1598–1640*, Brighton, Harvester, 1980

Patten, J., 'Patterns of migration and movement of labour to three pre-industrial East Anglian towns', *Journal of Historical Geography*, 2 (1976), 111–29

Patterson, A.T., *A History of Southampton 1700–1914*, Southampton, Southampton University Press, 1966

Pepys, *The Diary of Samuel Pepys*, eds R.C. Latham and W. Matthews, 11 vols, London, Bell & Hyman, 1970–83

——— *Letters and the Second Diary of Samuel Pepys*, ed. R.G. Howarth, London, Dent, 1933

Peter, Hugh, *Good Work for a Good Magistrate*, London, 1651

Petty, *The Economic Writings of Sir William Petty*, ed. C.H. Hull, 2 vols, Cambridge, Cambridge University Press, 1899

Pickering, D. (ed.), *The Statutes at Large*, vol. VII, London, 1763

Platt, C., *King Death. The Black Death and its aftermath in late-medieval England*, London, UCL Press, 1996

Plummer, A., *The London Weavers' Company 1600–1970*, London, Routledge & Kegan Paul, 1972

Porter, S., 'Death and burial in a London parish: St Mary Woolnoth 1653–99', *The London Journal*, 8 (1982), 76–80

———, *The Great Fire of London*, Stroud, Sutton, 1996

———, 'University and Society' in N. Tyacke (ed.), *The History of the University of Oxford, Volume IV, Seventeenth-Century Oxford*, Oxford, Clarendon Press, 1997

Power, M.J., 'The East and West in Early-Modern London', in E.W. Ives, R.J. Knecht and J.J. Scarisbrick (eds), *Wealth and Power in Tudor England* London, Athlone Press, 1978

———, 'The social topography of Restoration London', in A.L. Beier and R. Finlay (eds), *London 1500–1700: The making of the metropolis*

Priestley, U., 'The Norwich Textile Industry: The London Connection', *The London Journal*, 19 (1994), 108–18

Pullan, B., 'Plague and perceptions of the poor in early modern Italy', in T. Ranger and P. Slack (eds), *Epidemics and ideas: Essays on the historical perception of pestilence* Cambridge, Cambridge University Press, 1992

Race, P., 'Some further consideration of the Plague in Eyam 1665/6', *Local Population Studies*, 54 (1995), 56–65

Ranum, O., *Paris in the Age of Absolutism*, New York, John Wiley, 1968

Reed, M., 'Economic structure and change in seventeenth-century Ipswich' in P. Clark (ed.), *Country towns in pre-industrial England*

Reid, A. and Maniura, R. (eds), *Edward Alleyn: Elizabethan Actor, Jacobean Gentleman*, London, Dulwich Picture Gallery, 1994

Robertson, J.C., 'Reckoning with London: interpreting the *Bills of Mortality* before John Graunt', *Urban History*, 23 (1996), 325–50

Rosen, A., 'Winchester in transition, 1580–1700', in P. Clark (ed.), *Country towns in pre-industrial England*, Leicester, Leicester University Press, 1981

Rosen, G., *A History of Public Health*, Baltimore and London, John Hopkins University Press, 1993

Roseveare, H. (ed.), *Markets and Merchants of the Late Seventeenth Century: The Marescoe-David Letters, 1668–1680*, London, British Academy, Records of Social and Economic History, new series, 12, 1987

Roy, I., 'England turned Germany? The Aftermath of the Civil War in its European Context', *Transactions of the Royal Historical Society*, 5th series, 28 (1978), 127–44

——, 'Greenwich and the Civil War', *Transactions of the Greenwich and Lewisham Antiquarian Society*, 10 (1985), 12–20

——, 'The city of Oxford, 1640–60' in R.C. Richardson (ed.), *Town and Countryside in the English Revolution*, Manchester, Manchester University Press, 1992

RCHME, *Newark on Trent, the Civil War Siegeworks*, London, HMSO, 1964

Saunders, A. (ed.), *The Royal Exchange*, London Topographical Society, 152, 1997

Schama, S., *The Embarrassment of Riches. An Interpretation of Dutch Culture in the Golden Age*, London, Collins, 1987

Schove, D.J., 'Fire and Drought, 1600–1700', *Weather*, 21 (1966), 311–14

Schwoerer, L.G., *Lady Rachel Russell 'One of the Best of Women'*, Baltimore, John Hopkins University Press, 1988

Sheppard, F.H.W. (ed.), *Survey of London, Vol. 31, The Parish of St James, Westminster*, London, Athlone, 1963

Shrewsbury, J.F.D., *A History of Bubonic Plague in the British Isles*, Cambridge, Cambridge University Press, 1970

Sier, L.C., 'Experiences of the Great Fire of London, 1666', *Essex Review*, 51 (1942), 132–5

Slack, P., 'Books of Orders: the Making of English Social Policy, 1577–1631', *Transaction of the Royal Historical Society*, 5th series, 30 (1980), 1–22

——, 'The Disappearance of Plague: An Alternative View', *Economic History Review*, 34 (1981), 469–76

——, *The Impact of Plague in Tudor and Stuart England*, London, Routledge & Kegan Paul, 1985

——, 'Metropolitan government in crisis: the response to plague' in A.L. Beier and R. Finlay (eds), *London 1500–1700: The making of the metropolis*

Southey, Robert, *Letters from England*, ed. J. Simmons, Gloucester, Sutton, 1984

Spurr, J., '"Virtue, Religion and Government": the Anglican Uses of Providence', in T. Harris, P. Seaward and M. Goldie (eds), *The Politics of Religion in Restoration England* Oxford, Blackwell, 1990

——, *The Restoration Church of England, 1646–1689*, London and New Haven, Yale University Press, 1991

Sternberg, V.T., 'Predictions of the Fire and Plague of London', *Notes and Queries*, 1st series, 7 (1853), 79–80

Stocks, H. (ed.), *Records of the Borough of Leicester . . . , 1603–1688*, Cambridge, Cambridge University Press, 1923

Stoye, J., *Europe Unfolding, 1648–1688*, London, Collins, 1969

——, *English Travellers Abroad, 1604–1667*, 2nd edn, London and New Haven, Yale University Press, 1989

——, *Marsigli's Europe 1680–1730. The Life and Times of Luigi Ferdinando Marsigli, Soldier and Virtuoso*, New Haven and London, Yale University Press, 1994

Sutherland, I., 'When was the Great Plague? Mortality in London, 1563 to 1665' in D.V. Glass and R. Revelle (eds), *Population and Social Change* London, Arnold, 1972

Swift, Jonathan, *Journal to Stella*, ed. H. Williams, 2 vols, Oxford, Clarendon Press, 1948

Taswell, 'Autobiography and Anecdotes by William Taswell, D.D.', ed. G.P. Elliott, *Camden Miscellany*, vol. 2, 1853

Taylor, J., 'Plague in the towns of Hampshire: the Epidemic of 1665–6', *Southern History*, 6 (1984), 104–22

Tennant, P., *The Civil War in Stratford-upon-Avon. Conflict and Community in South Warwickshire, 1642–1646*, Stroud, Sutton, 1996

Thirsk, J. (ed.), *The Agrarian History of England and Wales, Volume V, 1640–1750: II. Agrarian Change*, Cambridge, Cambridge University Press, 1985

Thomas, J.H., *Town Government in the Sixteenth Century*, London, Allen & Unwin, 1933, reprinted, New York, Kelley, 1969

Thomas, K., *Religion and the Decline of Magic*, Harmondsworth, Penguin, 1973

Thomson, G.S., *Life in a Noble Household*, London, Cape, 1937

VCH, *Berkshire*, vol. 3, London, 1923

——, *Buckinghamshire*, vol. 3, London, 1925; vol. 4, London, 1927

——, *Cambridgeshire and the Isle of Ely*, vol. 3, London, 1959; vol. 4, London, 1953

——, *Essex*, vol. 9, London, 1994

——, *Gloucestershire*, vol. 4, 1988

——, *Lincolnshire*, vol. 2, London, 1906

——, *Middlesex*, vol. 9, London, 1989

——, *Staffordshire*, vol. 17, London, 1976

——, *Wiltshire*, vol. 5, London, 1957

Verney, F.P. and M.M., *Memoirs of the Verney Family during the Seventeenth Century*, 2nd edn, 2 vols, London, Longmans, Green, 1907

Wardale, J.R. (ed.), *Clare College Letters and Documents*, Cambridge, Macmillan & Bowes, 1903

West, R., *The Life & Strange Surprising Adventures of Daniel Defoe*, London, HarperCollins, 1997

Whiteway, William, *William Whiteway of Dorchester His Diary 1618 to 1635*, Dorset Record Society, vol. 12, 1991

Wills, C., *Plagues: Their Origins, History and Future*, London, HarperCollins, 1996

Wilson, F.P., *The Plague in Shakespeare's London*, Oxford, Clarendon Press, 1927

Winn, J.A., *John Dryden and His World*, New Haven and London, Yale University Press, 1987

Wrigley, E.A., 'A simple model of London's importance in changing English society and economy 1650–1750', *Past and Present*, 37 (1967), 44–70

—— and Schofield, R.S., *The Population History of England 1541–1871*, London, Arnold, 1981

Ziegler, P., *The Black Death*, Harmondsworth, Penguin, 1970

Zumthor, P., *Daily Life in Rembrandt's Holland*, Stanford, Stanford University Press, 1994

Index

Numbers in *italics* denote page numbers of illustrations